Understanding Psychology for Nursing Students

SAGE was founded in 1965 by Sara Miller McCune to support the dissemination of usable knowledge by publishing innovative and high-quality research and teaching content. Today, we publish over 900 journals, including those of more than 400 learned societies, more than 800 new books per year, and a growing range of library products including archives, data, case studies, reports, and video. SAGE remains majority-owned by our founder, and after Sara's lifetime will become owned by a charitable trust that secures our continued independence.

Los Angeles | London | New Delhi | Singapore | Washington DC | Melbourne

Understanding Psychology for Nursing Students

Jan De Vries and Fiona Timmins

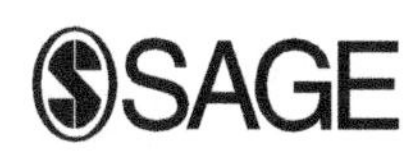

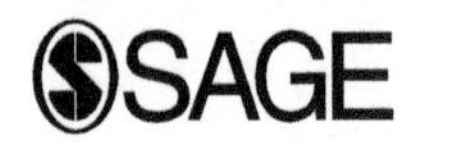
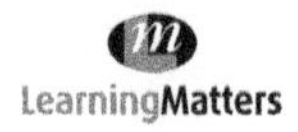

Learning Matters
An imprint of SAGE Publications Ltd
1 Oliver's Yard
55 City Road
London EC1Y 1SP

SAGE Publications Inc.
2455 Teller Road
Thousand Oaks, California 91320

SAGE Publications India Pvt Ltd
B 1/I 1 Mohan Cooperative Industrial Area
Mathura Road
New Delhi 110 044

SAGE Publications Asia-Pacific Pte Ltd
3 Church Street
#10-04 Samsung Hub
Singapore 049483

Library of Congress Control Number: 2016956882

British Library Cataloguing in Publication Data

A catalogue record for this book is available from the British Library.

ISBN 978-1-4129-6195-0 (pbk)
ISBN 978-1-4129-6194-3 (hbk)

Editor: Alex Clabburn
Development editor: Caroline Sheldrick
Production controller: Chris Marke
Project management: Deer Park Productions
Marketing manager: Tamara Navaratnam
Cover design: Wendy Scott
Typeset by: C&M Digitals (P) Ltd, Chennai, India
Printed in the UK

Contents

TRANSFORMING NURSING PRACTICE TNP

Transforming Nursing Practice is a series tailor-made for pre-registration student nurses. Each book in the series is:

- Affordable
- Mapped to the NMC Standards and Essential Skills Clusters
- Full of active learning features
- Focused on applying theory to practice

Each book addresses a core topic and has been carefully developed to be simple to use, quick to read and written in clear language.

"An invaluable series of books that explicitly relates to the NMC standards. Each book covers a different topic that students need to explore in order to develop into a qualified nurse... I would recommend this series to all pre-registration nursing students whatever their field or year of study

Linda Robson
Senior Lecturer, Edge Hill University

The set of books is an excellent resource for students. The series is small, easily portable and valuable. I use the whole set on a regular basis.

Fiona Davies
Senior Nurse Lecturer/Stage 1 Leader/Admissions Tutor, University of Derby

I recommend the SAGE/Learning Matters series to all my students as they are relevant and concise. Please keep up the good work.

Thomas Beary
Senior Lecturer in Mental Health Nursing, University of Hertfordshire"

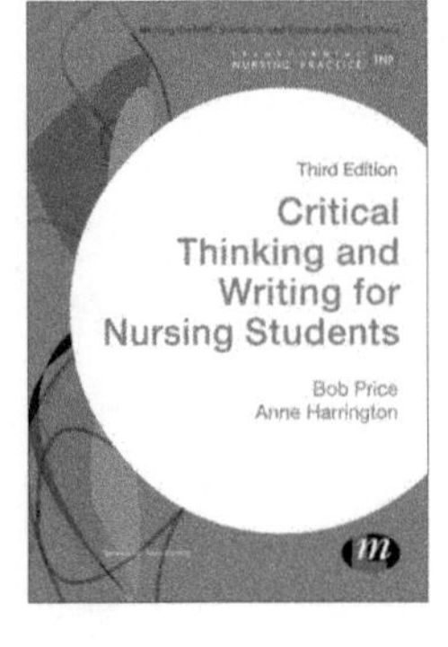

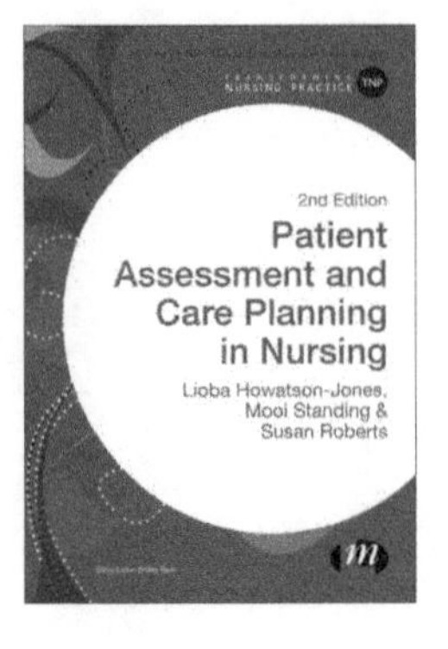

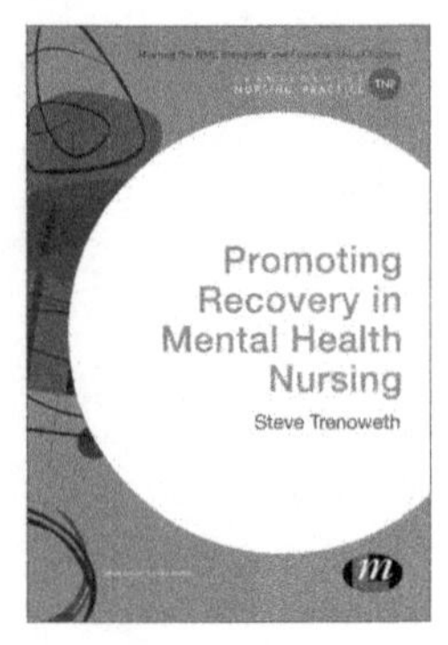

ABOUT THE SERIES EDITORS

Professor Shirley Bach is Head of the School of Health Sciences at the University of Brighton and responsible for the core knowledge titles. Previously she was head of post-graduate studies and has developed curriculum for undergraduate and pre-registration courses in a variety of subject domains.

Dr Mooi Standing is an Independent Academic Consultant (UK and International) and responsible for the personal and professional learning skills titles. She is an accredited NMC Quality Assurance Reviewer of educational programmes and a Professional Regulator Panellist on the NMC Practice Committee.

Sandra Walker is Senior Teaching Fellow in Mental Health at the University of Southampton and responsible for the mental health nursing titles. She is a Qualified Mental Health Nurse with a wide range of clinical experience spanning more than 20 years.

CORE KNOWLEDGE TITLES:

Becoming a Registered Nurse: Making the Transition to Practice
Communication and Interpersonal Skills in Nursing (3rd Ed)
Contexts of Contemporary Nursing (2nd Ed)
Getting into Nursing (2nd Ed)
Health Promotion and Public Health for Nursing Students (2nd Ed)
Introduction to Medicines Management in Nursing
Law and Professional Issues in Nursing (3rd Ed)
Leadership, Management and Team Working in Nursing (2nd Ed)
Learning Skills for Nursing Students
Medicines Management in Children's Nursing
Microbiology and Infection Prevention and Control for Nursing Students
Nursing and Collaborative Practice (2nd Ed)
Nursing and Mental Health Care
Nursing in Partnership with Patients and Carers
Palliative and End of Life Care in Nursing
Passing Calculations Tests for Nursing Students (3rd Ed)
Pathophysiology and Pharmacology for Nursing Students
Patient Assessment and Care Planning in Nursing (2nd Ed)
Patient Safety and Managing Risk in Nursing
Psychology and Sociology in Nursing (2nd Ed)
Successful Practice Learning for Nursing Students (2nd Ed)
Understanding Ethics in Nursing Students
Using Health Policy in Nursing Practice
What is Nursing? Exploring Theory and Practice (3rd Ed)

PERSONAL AND PROFESSIONAL LEARNING SKILLS TITLES:

Clinical Judgement and Decision Making for Nursing Students (2nd Ed)
Critical Thinking and Writing for Nursing Students (3rd Ed)
Evidence-based Practice in Nursing (3rd Ed)
Information Skills for Nursing Students
Reflective Practice in Nursing (3rd Ed)
Succeeding in Essays, Exams and OSCEs for Nursing Students
Succeeding in Literature Reviews and Research Project Plans for Nursing Students (2nd Ed)
Successful Professional Portfolios for Nursing Students (2nd Ed)
Understanding Research for Nursing Students (3rd Ed)

MENTAL HEALTH NURSING TITLES:

Assessment and Decision Making in Mental Health Nursing
Engagement and Therapeutic Communication in Mental Health Nursing
Medicines Management in Mental Health Nursing
Mental Health Law in Nursing
Physical Healthcare and Promotion in Mental Health Nursing
Promoting Recovery in Mental Health Nursing
Psychosocial Interventions in Mental Health Nursing

ADULT NURSING TITLES:

Acute and Critical Care in Adult Nursing (2nd Ed)
Caring for Older People in Nursing
Dementia Care in Nursing
Medicines Management in Adult Nursing
Nursing Adults with Long Term Conditions (2nd Ed)
Safeguarding Adults in Nursing Practice

About the authors

Jan de Vries works as an Assistant Professor at the School of Nursing and Midwifery, Trinity College Dublin. He completed his undergraduate and Masters studies at Utrecht University, Netherlands and his PhD at Trinity College Dublin, Ireland (1999). His teaching experience in psychology goes back over 30 years and includes the development, design and implementation of applied psychology modules and programmes in the Netherlands, Germany, Ireland, the UK and USA. He has lived in the Netherlands, Ireland and California and worked in several universities. He has also worked as a stress and trauma consultant, and coordinated programmes of dialogue at the Glencree Centre of Reconciliation in Ireland. He has been with the School of Nursing and Midwifery in Trinity College Dublin since 2007 and has worked tirelessly on developing the interface between psychology and nursing in a wide variety of contexts and at all relevant levels. This has included advising the Nursing and Midwifery Board of Ireland on psychology for nursing registration, curriculum development within Trinity College and a myriad of teaching modules at undergraduate and postgraduate level. His research interests include psychology of nursing, cognitive dissonance, mental health interventions, hand washing and several other health-care related topics. He has published reviews of a number of nursing psychology texts. Jan and Fiona have collaborated on several publications on the cusp of psychology and nursing.

Fiona Timmins works as an Associate Professor at the School of Nursing and Midwifery, Trinity College Dublin. In her role as a nurse academic she has published more than 100 publications in peer-reviewed journals and has written or co-authored seven nursing textbooks. She has presented widely internationally (more than 150 papers) including many Keynote presentations and workshops. She is currently one of the Editors of the *Journal of Nursing Management*, and acts as a reviewer for several peer-reviewed journals, sitting on the editorial board of many of these. Research interests include professional nursing issues, nurse education, spirituality and reflection. Her teaching skills were recognised in several awards including a Provost's Teaching Award in 2004 (**http://www.tcd.ie/CAPSL/awards/provost/archive/#PTA2005**). She has several degrees and awards including a PhD in nursing from the University of Glamorgan.

Sources and acknowledgements

The authors and publisher wish to thank the following for permission to reproduce copyright material:

American Scientist Magazine, for material adapted from Plutchik, R. (1980). *Emotion: A psychoevolutionary synthesis*, forming Figure 6.4: Primary Emotions.

McGraw-Hill Education (UK) for material taken from Ogden, J. (2012). *Health psychology*, forming Figure 9.2 Leventhal's Self-regulatory model of illness behaviour, and Figure 9.3: Coping with the Crisis of Illness, Moos and Schaefer model (1984);

Taylor & Francis Ltd for material adapted from Stroebe, M. and Schut, H. (1999), p. 213. The dual process model of coping with bereavement: rationale and description. *Death Studies*, 23: 197–224, forming Figure 9.6: Dual process of coping with bereavement.

Introduction

Psychology has long been an integral component of nursing education curricula internationally. Even early nursing sources argue that psychology is indispensable to the nurse in understanding the patients, advancing their treatment effectively, and to understand themselves and their colleagues. Indeed psychology as a distinct subject has been gaining increasing relevance within the nursing curriculum over the last 50 years, with burgeoning texts on the topic reflecting a continuously growing awareness of its importance. Considering the progress in both nursing and psychology it stands to reason that there is a need for up-to date nursing psychology texts to capture this development. This text has been written with this in mind.

This book is intended for nursing students throughout their education and registered nurses who like to upgrade their knowledge and skills. It provides an innovative and practical perspective on the role of contemporary psychology in nursing, with reference to progress in each field as well as common problem areas. Great effort has been put into presenting the material in an accessible and understandable way to ensure that the reader will remain captivated and engaged. Written by a psychologist and a nurse who both work in nursing education, the emphasis has been on ensuring that this book speaks to nurses. Years of experience has helped the authors to get to the point quickly and avoid overly laborious explanations and detail.

For the nurse educator it is important to know that the text provides many activities to engage the students in an active way. This will be of considerable help in designing learning modules, interactive sessions, lectures and workshops. Moreover, the text is designed to facilitate problem-based and enquiry-based learning and includes self-directed and web-based learning assignments. In some nursing schools today psychology is taught as a distinct topic, in many others it is integrated within nursing modules. This text has been designed for use within both contexts. Its focus is not only on understanding and using psychology within nursing, but also to apply and integrate it in practical nursing and health care.

The text has been designed to be as relevant for general nurses in hospitals, as for community or public health nurses, mental health nurses, children's nurses, and intellectual disability nurses. Moreover, it addresses the psychological requirements for nurse registration in the United Kingdom (NMC 2010) and the Republic of Ireland (NMBI 2016) and presents relevant theory and research, as well as psychological tools and skills that are integral to care provision in Europe. In particular the UK Nursing and Midwifery Council (NMC) requirements are carefully integrated in the text.

The NMC (2010:7) identifies knowledge, skills and attitudes that nursing students are obliged to acquire during their preparatory educational programme. Four domains are outlined which relate to competencies that nursing students need to develop during their education. Each domain includes several competencies of which many, although not explicitly stated, are informed by psychology. This book provides both fundamental content at the basis of the competencies in each domain and specific support for the development of the practical skills involved.

How this book corresponds with NMC educational requirements for nurse registration:

- *Domain 1: Professional values (NMC 2010: 13-14)*
  Several core aspects within this domain are addressed. In a general sense, the call for a 'holistic, non-judgemental, caring and sensitive manner' in care (competency 2) is responded to throughout the text by providing a psychological framework for understanding how this is achieved and which obstacles are encountered. Specifically, working in partnership, health and wellness promotion, and how to maintain the dignity of patients (competencies 3 and 4) are developed in Chapters 1, 2, 8, 9 and 10. Also, fostering 'reflection' (competency 8) is essential throughout the text, as is the appreciation of 'the value of evidence in practice' (competency 9) Furthermore, core factors in how to improve nursing performance and safety (competency 7) are presented in Chapters 4, 5, 6, and 7.
- *Domain 2: Communication and interpersonal skills (NMC 2010: 15-16)*
  Psychology contributes in a generic way to the development of communication and interpersonal skills. Every chapter in this book is aimed at promoting the development of these skills through the included activities. In Chapters 1, 9, and 10 particular attention is paid to the development of person-centred care (competency 2) and the obstacles nurses encounter to practice in this way. In Chapters 1, 4, 8 and 9 the focus is on how different psychological approaches can be used in optimising communication to reduce stress and anxiety (competency 4) and encourage health-promotion and recovery (competency 6). The text specifically helps nurses to 'recognise when people are anxious or in distress and respond effectively, using therapeutic principles' (competency 4). This is done by identifying and applying principles of humanistic, behavioural, cognitive and positive psychology, and translating these into therapeutic principles in nursing.
- *Domain 3: Nursing practice and decision making (NMC 2010: 17-19)*
  Making safe decisions based on evidence and sound assessment (competency 1) requires an understanding of cognitive strengths and limitations in information processing. This is addressed in Chapters 5 and 6. Moreover the text (in particular Chapter 2, 3, 5, and 8) presents practical 'knowledge of the structure and functions of the human body, and other relevant knowledge from the life, behavioural and social sciences as applied to health, ill health, disability, ageing and death' (competency 2). How to provide educational support and ensure self-care in patients and families (competency 8) is addressed in Chapter 4 and 9. The importance and particulars of how to evaluate one's care levels (competency 10) is addressed specifically in Chapter 10.

- *Domain 4: Leadership, management and team working (NMC 2010:20-21)*
Much of the emphasis of the book is on understanding social factors in collaboration with colleagues and multi-disciplinary teams in health care organisations. In particular Chapter 7 provides a foundation for developing this domain. Throughout the text it is the ambition of the authors to further cultivate the role of nurses as 'change agents' (competency 1). Of the other competencies included in this domain, how to ensure 'systematic evaluation of care' (competency 2) is emphasised in Chapter 10. Finally, 'self-awareness' (competency 4) is a general aim of the text and specifically emphasised in Chapters 2, 3 and 6, while working in teams and how to optimise one's ability to do so is included in Chapter 7.

While this is a concise text, its scope is ambitious. It is our belief that psychology has much to offer to nurses. Therefore, in addition to a foundation in psychology, the emphasis is on its application and integration in care provision. Though the chapters are constructed to be understood separately, they also build on one another. Three introductory chapters (Ch 1-3) are followed by four specific topic areas and their nursing applications (Ch 4-7) and culminate in the integration of psychology in nursing care (Ch 8-10). Key themes are presented in ways that allow the reader to relate, reflect and exercise in order to build up a meaningful well-structured and practical knowledge base around the psychology of nursing and health care. This book also aims to get the reader to question their understanding of nursing care and challenge issues that compromise practice and quality of care.

Anyone who has been a patient in a hospital or received care in a different context remembers those nurses who were particularly helpful and understanding, were prepared to go the extra mile, or were unique in their ability to anticipate the needs of patients. Even years later, this might come up in conversation. Their names may not be remembered, but it is clear that these nurses made a real difference. This book aspires to assist students and practitioners to become one of them!

References

NMC (2010). Standards of proficiency for pre-registration nursing education. London: Nursing and Midwifery Council (http://www.nmc-uk.org/documents/standards/nmcstandardsofproficiencyforpre_registrationnursingeducation.pdf)

NMBI (2016). Requirements and Standards for Nurse Registration Education Programmes (4th ed). Dublin: Nursing and Midwifery Board of Ireland.
http://www.nmbi.ie/Education/Standards-and-Requirements/Nurse-Registration-Programmes

Chapter 1
Psychology as a field of study and why nurses need to know about it

Chapter aims

After reading this chapter you will be able to:

- explain what psychology is and how it applies and contributes to nursing;
- consider psychological aspects in a variety of health-care and nursing situations;
- outline how psychologists do research and how to apply psychological research methods to nursing and health-care problems;
- discuss how psychology fits into the bio-psycho-social model.

This chapter introduces the field of psychology, demonstrating how psychology teaches us to reflect on behaviour and mental processes in both ourselves and in other people. We will look at how psychology informs our knowledge of the non-medical aspects of health and illness. The chapter introduces you to a psychological mind-set that will inform your provision of care, and provides a background knowledge that will help in your lifelong learning. Every step of the way you will see the relevance of psychology to nursing and health care. If you are ambitious to make a difference in your discipline, psychology can be a real asset. Ask patients and families, even years later, to give an account of their experiences in health care, and they invariably remember the nurse who provided more than expert care, also offering warmth, hope, intelligent support and inspiration. This book is intended to assist you in becoming that nurse!

While we recognise that you may refer to people in your care in different ways, such as 'patient', 'client', or 'service user', we will refer to them mostly as 'patients' for the sake of simplicity. 'Patient/client/service user' is a bit awkward, don't you agree?

Introduction

What is psychology?

Psychology is often defined as the '**scientific study of behaviour and mental processes**' (Nolen-Hoeksema *et al.*, 2014, p. 5). Thus it focuses not only on what we do, and how and why we do it, but also on our feelings, our thinking and everything else that goes on in our heads. Since much of what we do, feel and think is related to other humans, psychology also focuses on our relationships and interactions with others. If we want to make sure that we don't exclude anything from how we define psychology, it would be perfectly acceptable to consider it the study of the human experience. The term 'scientific' suggests that psychology is more than using our powers of observation, interpretation and reasoning to make sense of ourselves and others. Psychologists also make use of systematic methods of research and gather and evaluate evidence to test any statement made about the human experience.

Because psychology is about us, it has been widely applied for practical use in areas such as education, media, architecture, city planning, manufacturing, retail, etc. It also has a firm foothold in other sciences such as business studies, economics, anthropology, sociology and engineering. Relevant for you, psychology has practical applications to nursing and health care and contributes theoretically and in research to our understanding of health, illness, medicine and nursing theory. The next section will give you an impression of these applications and how they are approached within this book.

Why should nurses learn about psychology?

The short answer to this question is that regulating bodies for nursing education prescribe the inclusion of psychology to become a registered nurse (see the Introduction of this book). The long answer is in this book. Every step of the way we will apply psychology to nursing and health care and, hopefully, it will become and remain clear to you why it is useful. We'll highlight some important reasons below.

The importance of psychology was recognised even at the beginning of the twentieth century when both fields were still in their infancy as subjects of scholarly study. An early author of a psychology text for nursing phrased the future of psychology in nursing in urgent terms:

> *The time will come inevitably, when all training schools of standing will include the subject in the course of study, and, as a result, the power of nursing will increase immeasurably. A large proportion of nurses' blunders occur because they do not possess a working knowledge of psychology. Psychology should not be considered a subject which may be included in the nursing curriculum, but as one which cannot be omitted.*
>
> (Higgins, 1921, p. vii.)

More broadly, the nursing literature identified psychology as important, in particular because of its practical use in helping nurses understand themselves, the care they provide, the people in their care, their colleagues, and the health-care organisations and communities within which they work (de Vries and Timmins, 2012). Ultimately this is aimed at optimising care.

Let us see if we can make this come alive for you. In the next section we'll present a series of scenarios that relate to practical nursing situations and problems. This will elucidate the application of psychology while also providing an overview of what you will learn in this book.

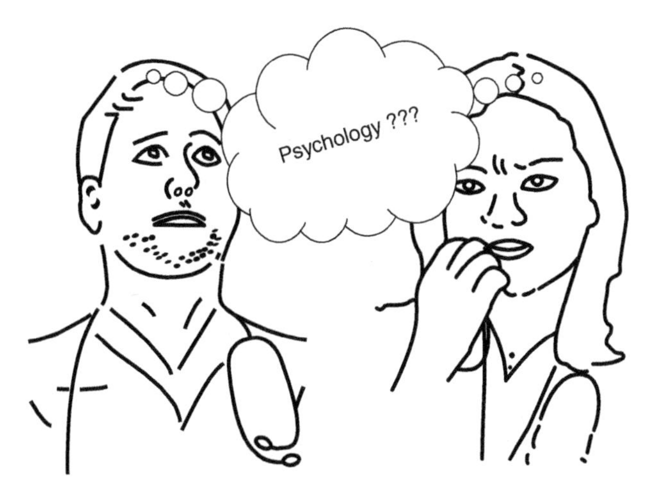

Figure 1.1: Why should nurses study psychology?

The application of psychology in nursing

Place yourself in the role of the nurse, reflect on each of the situations and try to answer the questions. Don't worry if it is not immediately clear to you what each scenario is about. You may want to turn to the chapters indicated to preview the content.

Scenario: Making contact (*see* Chs 2 and 10)

Someone in your care is uncommunicative and looks sad. Your questions meet with very short answers and the person does not look you in the eyes. You feel that it is important to get through to her because there are decisions to be made that require the person's active contribution. Intuitively what approach would you take and what are the alternatives?

Relevant themes: different schools of thought within psychology.

An outline response is provided at the end of the chapter.

Nurses often make intuitive decisions about how to communicate but, as a professional, it is important to understand why you do what you do so you can develop it further and become really good at it. Psychology offers assistance and background to make informed choices and practical guidance to enhance communication between nurse and patient. In this case, different psychological perspectives or schools of thought indicate a variety of approaches to be taken. Chapters 2 and 10 will provide considerations on, for instance, offering effective emotional support (humanistic), help with decision making (cognitive), providing encouragement (behavioural) and giving positive energy (positive psychology).

Scenario: Understanding the brain (*see* Ch. 3)

In a team meeting a neurologist explains how one of the patients who had a serious car accident has suffered lesions in the brain. There is clear evidence of damage to the hindbrain (cerebellum), but the results are less clear on how subcortical areas such as the amygdala and hypothalamus are affected. When asked about your observations of the patient in the last few days you are not sure what to say. Without knowing what to look for you did not really pay that much attention. Can you argue why it is important for a nurse to be able to discuss these matters with a doctor?

Relevant themes: structure and functions of the nervous system and the brain; sensation and perception.

An outline response is provided at the end of the chapter.

Psychologists emphasise that the way in which people function cannot be appreciated if we don't study how it is organised in the brain and nervous system. Psychology and biology overlap here. Chapter 3 is specifically aimed at helping nurses grasp how the structure and functions of the brain relate and how this is expressed in what you see in the people in your care. This will allow you to communicate and contribute to team meetings in which matters of the brain are discussed. In regard to this scenario, if you had, for instance, perceived uncontrolled emotional outbursts in the patient, you would have realised that these would have been relevant to the consultant's query (because they would suggest the amygdala could be affected).

Scenario: Development and learning (see Ch. 4)

As part of your daily routine you are instructing patients of different ages in several ways (to use crutches, sort medication, eat independently, recognise triggers for becoming unwell, health promotion, etc.). After a while you start to realise that your approach is different for various age groups. Moreover, it transpires that individuals learn in very different ways. Can you give examples of age differences in learning?

Relevant themes: stages of development and approaches to learning.

An outline response is provided at the end of the chapter.

Without comprehension of the complexity of developmental and learning processes it is going to be very hard to teach even simple things. Also, your efforts to affect the thinking, emotions and behaviour of the people in your care will be hit and miss. Reading Chapter 4 will help you to fathom these processes and apply them in multiple ways. Learning will be more effective if you take experience and development into account, identify the readiness to learn a specific skill or principle, and ascertain what kind of support needs to be provided. Association, encouragement, modelling and understanding are part of many learning experiences. Psychology provides the foundation of how to support and influence the people in your care.

Scenario: Nightshift (see Chs 5 and 6)

You have just started the third night of a nightshift. You had a little difficulty sleeping during the last couple of days. Your mind is a bit clouded. You misjudge a situation because you jumped to a conclusion. You are physically fine, but find it hard to focus. You realise that there are some gaps in your memory of your shift. How should you address this situation?

Relevant themes: consciousness, sleep, memory.

An outline response is provided at the end of the chapter.

Chapter 5 will provide you with an outline of how memory and consciousness work, including sleep processes and issues that can arise, thus helping you to understand why the lack of sleep has affected your judgement and memory. Based on this you might like then to plan ways to improve your sleep effectiveness. Irregular hours and shift work are commonplace in nursing and it is important that you begin to understand and develop ways to deal with changing patterns of sleep so that you remain at all times a safe and effective practitioner.

Scenario: Under pressure (see Ch. 6)

You are on duty in a busy Emergency Department (ED). Tensions are rising because people have to wait much longer than they had hoped for. There is a lot of complaining. Consequently, you are put under pressure and find it hard to keep making rational decisions about care priorities. At the end of the night you are in turmoil. Even when you arrive home you are still trying to defend to yourself why you made some decisions. Would you consider yourself a conscientious nurse in this situation?

Relevant themes: understanding of thinking, motivation, emotions.

An outline response is provided at the end of the chapter.

Your understanding of why you might feel in turmoil in such a situation is greatly helped by recognising the psychological mechanisms whereby your inner peace gets disrupted. It also helps to be aware of how we may slip from rational into sloppy and simplistic thinking. These mechanisms are addressed in Chapter 6. Being aware of these processes does not mean you are no longer affected by them, but at least you can warn yourself and prevent a debacle. The general focus of Chapter 6 is on thinking, motivation and emotion and hits at the core of the skills nurses need to develop to be effective in their care.

Scenario: Group influence (see Ch. 7)

You are working together in a new team and are reflecting on why you interacted with the people in your care just like your new colleagues did. Not that there was anything wrong with it, but still there were a few aspects you had learned differently. The next day the whole group reverts to the approach that you had learned while a supervisor is present. This puzzles you. You also note that safety protocols are followed more rigidly that day. What are the positives and negatives of what you observed?

Relevant themes: understanding of social interaction, social influence, conformity, obedience, working in a large health-care organisation.

An outline response is provided at the end of the chapter.

This scenario illustrates the impact of conformity or group pressure on the first day, and the impact of obedience on the second day. Social psychologists have done revealing and shocking research on these topics, which serve as a stark warning for all who work with other people. Chapter 7 looks at all main aspects of social interaction partly to assist you in becoming effective in how you collaborate and interact with others, and partly to ensure that you appreciate the power of the social situation in large health-care institutions.

Scenario: Stress (see Ch. 8)

Since the new management took over in the hospital, things are not the same. Cost cutting has led to lay-offs, longer hours, and a new system of shifts has been introduced. Average sick days per month among staff have doubled and the department you work in is threatened with closure. Nobody knows exactly what is going to happen. You are worried about the care you can provide. Relationships between you and your colleagues are tense. What can you do?

Relevant themes: stress and health, stress management.

An outline response is provided at the end of the chapter.

Health and stress are important matters of interest for everyone. This includes people who work under pressure, such as nurses. Many of you will find yourselves working for large health-care organisations where perpetual change, funding and staffing issues are common. While it is important to know what keeps you healthy in general, it becomes particularly urgent to know what to do and what to avoid when you are experiencing long-term stress. The most worrying aspect in the scenario is that 'average sick days have doubled'. Once you've read Chapter 8 you will fully appreciate why this is so. You will also comprehend more fully why psychologists are interested in nutrition and exercise, and why remaining positive is helpful (*see also* Chapters 6 and 10).

Scenario: Illness as a crisis (*see* Ch. 9)

Many of your patients experience being in the hospital as a crisis, but not always in the way you would expect. One man tells you that he is much less worried about himself than about how his small company will fare in his absence. His visiting hours look like business meetings. He seems worn out and in pain, but should you rescue him by sending his business partner away?

Relevant themes: crisis of illness.

An outline response is provided at the end of the chapter.

As a nurse, you tend to experience patients only in the health-care setting, but not at home or at work. As a result your insight into the overall impact of their condition may be limited. Psychologists would argue that it is essential to appreciate the whole situation around the person in order to provide the best care. Chapter 9 addresses the crisis of illness in order to enhance not just your appreciation of this, but also to instruct you in the most common ways in which crises impact people in health care. We address the psychology of chronic illness, pain, chronic fatigue, mental health problems, stigma, loss and grief. Psychology deepens the understanding of the way in which these issues affect the people in your care.

Scenario: Person-centred versus task-oriented nursing (see Ch. 10)

Nurse A *listens, shows empathy, takes time with each patient and family, expresses an interest in both the patient and family, and involves them in all decisions.*

Nurse B *works efficiently, has her work done on time, instructs and advises patients, and avoids invading the privacy between patient and family.*

What are the strengths and weaknesses of each approach?

Relevant themes: psychology of care, principles of psychology and their practical implications for care.

An outline response is provided at the end of the chapter.

You will most likely suggest that Nurse A will have more success and from your readings in Chapter 10, you will find out that this is correct. Overall, treating patients in a way that is person-centred and shows an interest is more likely to build the good relationships that are a vehicle for effective care and support. It is also likely that both the patient and family will have a better care experience. It is important for you to know that many aspects of effective care are rooted in psychology. Chapter 10 is the accumulation of this and seeks to outline the implications for care provision, with reference to all common nursing tasks. After reading this highly practical chapter you should be able to apply and further develop principles of psychology in your care.

Activity 1.1 *Reflection*

Think about the scenarios presented and reflect on each of the questions. Preview the relevant chapters to explore the content for cues. Discussing it with other students will add an important dimension.

An outline response is provided at the end of the chapter.

We will introduce many more scenarios, case studies and activities in the book. These are essential to the active learning experience we advocate. Beginning the reflective process will also be important for you, as it will help you to connect your life experience and experience from your nursing course with the content of this book. Looking at the concepts early on in your reading will be useful, because you will think about them and they will begin to distil in your mind. Later on when you revisit the chapters you will find the reading and learning easier, more familiar and you will be better able to apply it. You may find that you have already started to add to your insight simply by thinking about the issues raised.

Besides psychology's contribution to addressing nursing problems, an important consideration at this point is that the two fields (nursing and psychology) have in common ethical principles for the provision of care. In the practice of both professional fields, there is an obligation to conduct oneself with respect, and to demonstrate competence, responsibility and integrity. In the professional practice of psychology you must be 'open, honest and transparent, accountable, evidence based and inclusive' (BPS, 2015) and this level of ethical practice is also reflected in UK nursing guidelines (NMC, 2010). It is safe to say that the 'do no harm' principle is as ingrained in psychological care as it is in nursing.

The bio-psycho-social model

In your efforts to make sense of the scenarios in this chapter you will most likely have noticed that your thoughts will not have been confined to the domain of psychology. It is likely that you will have simultaneously considered medical or biological aspects, and psychological and social aspects of care such as family, community and ethnic background. That is because they are interconnected. This principle of interconnectedness is the basis of contemporary health care.

Bio-psycho-social (see Figure 1.1) thinking is essential for good nursing. We'll come back to this in Chapter 8 when we look at Health Psychology but, for now, let us just make sure that you understand how important it is. Of course nurses are perhaps first concerned with physical health. Is the patient recovering physically? What are the physical or biological signs (blood pressure, breathing, signs of infection, alertness, sleep, etc.)? But you should also be interested in the patient's mood, emotions and thinking about the illness, the motivation to get better and other psychological

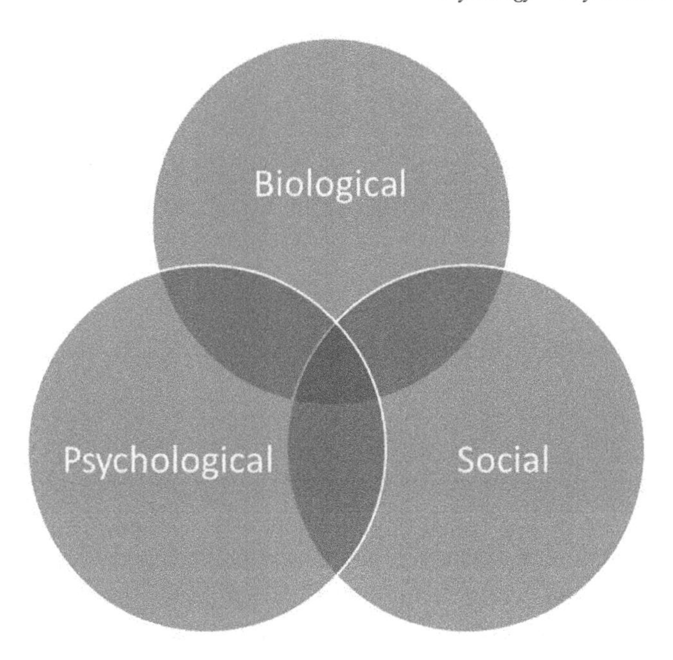

Figure 1.2: The bio-psycho-social model

factors. Beyond the personal aspect you will consider whether whoever visits provides the patient with social support and, perhaps, the broader impact of family, community and society. Together this generates a 'holistic' perspective. Likewise you will look at the care you provide, again, perhaps, first in a physical sense: am I contributing to helping the patient physically? However, you would like to see that you have contributed to psychological factors such as mood improvement, reduced stress, or a more upbeat outlook on the future. Furthermore, you will have considered social aspects of your care such as recruiting family in the provision of optimal support to the patient and preparing a pathway to returning to work and other social commitments.

Activity 1.2 — *Reflection*

Discuss how the three factors in the bio-psycho-social model are involved in these interactions with people in your care.

	Biological	**Psychological**	**Social**
a. Taking blood pressure			
b. Listening to someone who is upset			
c. Discussing hospital discharge and support at home			
d. Giving a patient a bedpan			
e. Helping a child understand her condition			
f. Organising a group activity with people in your care			

An outline response is provided at the end of the chapter.

What do psychologists do?

Thus far the main focus in this chapter has been on demonstrating the relevance of psychology to nursing and explaining its place in the bio-psycho-social model of health care. In the remainder of this chapter we put the psychologist as a professional and a researcher in the spotlight. As you will see, this simultaneously creates an opportunity to demonstrate how psychological research takes place in health care and nursing.

Psychologists as professionals

One of the common misconceptions about psychologists is that they are all involved in providing psychotherapy. The term 'psychologist' is often equated with psychotherapist and, while it is true that many psychologists are therapists, you find them employed in numerous other positions too. These include, of course, the role of educator or researcher – we've already mentioned this – but they are also working as advisors within organisations and companies. They work in communities, government, television networks, manufacturing, aviation, the police force, military, prison, supermarkets, and also in hospitals. Psychologists can be found in almost any industry and type of activity, because they have studied humans in detail to a degree that no other field of study does.

Psychologists bring a depth of thinking and analysis to the table that is valued in many different situations. Furthermore, psychologists have often specialised in particular types of activity or industry. Thus a psychologist who has concentrated on organisational psychology may be working for a large company. A psychologist who has focused on consumer behaviour may find that a supermarket chain is interested in his or her services. In health care, we would perhaps be most interested in what a health psychologist can contribute and it should not surprise us then that many health-care centres employ health psychologists. It is the awareness of fundamental principles and mechanisms in human behaviour, thinking and emotions that makes psychologists much sought after. As we will see, it is not only health psychology but, rather, a wide variety of principles of psychology that are applicable to health care and therefore also to nursing. This book offers the application of a broad basis of psychological knowledge and skills to enable nurses to think a bit like a psychologist and to integrate this thinking within clinical practice.

Activity 1.3 — *Reflection*

Do you ever operate with a psychological mind-set? Let's take the test.

Choose between never (0), sometimes (1) and regularly (2) in response to the following ten statements. Try to be honest. Add up your score at the end.

	never	sometimes	regularly
1. I am curious about other people's thoughts	0	1	2
2. I try to find out what might help people	0	1	2
3. I wonder why I feel the way I do	0	1	2

4.	I say things to make others feel good	0	1	2
5.	I think and talk about relationships	0	1	2
6.	I read about psychological topics	0	1	2
7.	I analyse problems of humanity	0	1	2
8.	Friends come to me for emotional support	0	1	2
9.	I make an effort to manage my stress	0	1	2
10.	I do my best to resolve conflict	0	1	2

You will have noted that the above statements are related to reflection and possessing an interest in understanding oneself and others, and the application of psychology to helping ourselves and others. These are core aims of psychology. If you have scored more than 10 points in this test you are already frequently using a psychological mind-set in your daily life, even if you are not aware of this. If you scored between 5-10 points you likely do so every now and again. If you scored less than 5 points you may at present not use a psychological outlook that often. Perhaps reading about psychology will change this.

An outline response is provided at the end of the chapter.

How do psychologists do research?

The knowledge, mechanisms and principles introduced in this book have all emerged as a result of empirical research. We've already pointed out that research is at the core of the development of the field, but how is it done? To answer this question we will look first at the general process of research in psychology, followed by the specific methods used.

The research process in psychology

- *Observation:*
  Almost all research starts with the first-hand observation of phenomena in the world. In psychology these phenomena are inevitably related to human activity, experiences and interactions of people and their environment. What we observe is affected by our interests, expectations and understanding. It is limited by what we can be aware of.

- *Identify questions, problems, issues:*
  The next step is essential to the psychological mind-set. Psychologists will look for aspects that we have difficulty understanding, and will point out problems or issues that are worth addressing. This requires a critical perspective and a tendency to ask questions and take nothing for granted. Psychologists zone in on issues of fundamental interest as well as problems that are important for society.

- *Suggest a way of understanding them:*
  With each identified issue, what is presently known about it will be scrutinized and efforts will be made to come to an understanding. If we are not sure, which is often the case, the understanding of the phenomenon will be proposed as a hypothesis – an educated

guess about cause and effect. Our way of understanding will be affected by what we already know, theories and previously acquired scientific evidence. However, it is also possible that we stumble upon more than one possible explanation, or we may find ourselves puzzled because none of the known theories apply.

- *Gathering systematic evidence:*
  If we have developed a hypothesis, our focus will be on testing that hypothesis in an empirical research study. It is essential that we set up such a study in an unbiased way. This means that we are equally open to establishing evidence in support of or against the hypothesis. If we have not developed a hypothesis our research efforts may be of an exploratory nature, which can in future lead to the development of hypotheses. The research methods psychologists use are discussed in the next section.
- *Publishing results:*
  There is no point in performing research if the results are not publicised. It is essential that the scientific community, but also the general public, learn about the findings of a study. Generally, psychologists would seek to publish their findings in credible journals that subscribe to a process known as peer-review. This means that a panel of peers, who specialise in the specific area of the study, establish whether the method and procedure of the study were reliable and valid. This is a protective process that is intended to prevent the publication of flawed scientific evidence, which would obscure rather than enlighten our understanding of a specific issue. Psychological findings of wider public interest are usually picked up by popular psychology books and magazines, websites, newspapers and other media. This is really important because, in this way, psychological knowledge spreads throughout society and can benefit us all.
- *Theory building:*
  Theory based on sound empirical evidence is the desired outcome of any research process. It is a dialectic process, which may spread across decades or even centuries and which may involve the efforts of hundreds of researchers. Sometimes a specific theory is in vogue and inspires continuous empirical effort. Sometimes theories are supported for ideological or political reasons. Some topics may be taboo. Funding plays an important role in deciding which theories are investigated and which are left to lie dormant. Of course, this affects scientific progress and brings bias into theory building. In a way, it is perhaps more honest to say that the research process attempts to be scientific and unbiased, but does not always succeed in this. Psychology has a history of hotly debated theories that were sometimes falsified after having been supported for long periods of time. Think of the turbulent history of how the understanding of our planet and solar system (Galileo and Copernicus) evolved. The development of psychological theory is not very different!

Research methods

Research is often divided into qualitative and quantitative methods (Polit and Beck, 2013). **Quantitative research** emphasises finding out about the magnitude of a phenomenon whereas **qualitative research** focuses on understanding the features and identity of a phenomenon. Sometimes research is done using a combination of quantitative and qualitative approaches. This is called mixed-methods research. Nurses need to know about the principles of research in order to critically read research papers and to be able to engage in research themselves (NMC, 2015).

Activity 1.4 *Evidence-based practice and research*

Quantitative vs. qualitative research

Hospital management wants to learn about patients' satisfaction with their stay in a hospital. Researchers have proposed the following approaches.

Quantitative approach

On a scale from 0 (not at all satisfied) to 10 (very highly satisfied) could you indicate how satisfied you are with your stay in our hospital? (Please circle the number that best represents your level of satisfaction.)

0 1 2 3 4 5 6 7 8 9 10

Qualitative approach

Can you tell us whether you are satisfied with your stay in the hospital? Please explain why or why not in the box below!

Discuss the advantages and disadvantages of the two research approaches.

An outline response is provided at the end of the chapter.

Research in psychology as well as in nursing tends to make use of several approaches. We'll discuss them here.

Naturalistic observation

This type of study involves observation of behaviour and interaction between people in their natural environment. This approach has long been used to study animal behaviour, but it is also suitable for studying human behaviour. You can, for instance, observe nurse, patient or visitor behaviour in hospitals. In the past, such research often made use of checklists to record observed behaviours. Today, cameras or audio recording equipment allow for repeated and more detailed analysis. The use of CCTV has further expanded the possibilities, although the ethical considerations are a significant issue in these types of studies.

Interviews

Interviews typically make use of questions to elicit information regarding issues of interest to the research team. The questions may be wide open ('can you tell us your opinion on health?') or specifically focused ('is your chronic condition a concern for you or not?'). The interview may involve a meeting between interviewer and interviewee or it may take place on the phone or even online. Sometimes group interviews or focus groups are used to elicit the opinions of several people at the same time. Generally, interviews are recorded and the recording is transcribed. These days, researchers tend to make use of data management programmes and a wide variety of data analysis methods (Denzin and Lincoln, 2011).

Case Study

The detailed study of one person or one situation is a case study. A study that a doctor made of the whole history of treatment of a specific patient is a case study. But so is the study of a hospital in which problems occurred that required investigating. A case study often provides extensive detail, often from different sources. Case studies were particularly popular in the early development of psychology.

Surveys

Surveys or questionnaires generally consist of a list of pre-coded questions that are distributed by mail, accessible online or asked in person or over the phone. The questions usually require responses on a series of scales (see Activity 1.4) or a choice of different answer categories. They can be short or very detailed and long. A census is usually conducted in the form of a survey and so are opinion polls.

Correlational studies

This type of study does not have to involve gathering new data. The data may already be available. Hospitals document the type of conditions or illnesses, mortality rates, length of hospital stay, and many demographic aspects such as age and gender. This makes it possible to find out what the relationship or correlation is between these factors or variables. You could establish what the mortality rates are for specific conditions over the years and see if there is a difference for men and women. You could also find out which conditions lead to the longest hospital admissions. Health psychologists have made use of the behavioural data GPs gather (such as exercise habits, smoking and diet) to establish the relationship between these factors and certain illnesses. However, beware, because finding a correlation does not mean that we've figured out which causes which.

Experiments

Experimental studies (see Useful websites at the end of this chapter) have provided some of the most interesting and talked-about findings within psychology. In an experiment 'the investigator manipulates a variable *(independent)* under carefully controlled conditions and observes whether any changes occur in a second variable *(dependent)* as a result' (Weiten, 2010, p. 40). We distinguish between lab experiments, which take place under carefully controlled conditions in which a limited number of dependent variables are manipulated to measure their effect on an outcome or dependent variables, and field experiments, which use the same principles but they take place in a natural environment and participants may not be aware they are part of an experiment. In quasi-experiments the independent variable is naturally occurring, so there is no manipulation, but the impact of the variation on a dependent variable is measured.

Concept summary: Lab, field and quasi-experiment

All three of these approaches could be used to test the impact of the two nursing approaches in the Scenario: Person-Centred versus Task-Oriented Nursing – person-centred Care with Nurse A *versus* task-oriented care Nurse B (see page 7).

If we did it as a **lab experiment** we might use a lab environment with mock patients who would receive one type of nursing on one day and another type of nursing on another day. If we carefully instruct all nurses in roles A and B they can alternate the care approach they portray. The mock patients would provide satisfaction ratings at regular intervals.

As a **field experiment**, we would do the same except in a real hospital with real patients.

As a **quasi-experiment** we would not instruct nurses but rate them on their natural inclinations on the person-centred *versus* task-oriented dichotomy and ask patients to express their satisfaction on a rating scale after repeated exposure to each nurse.

Discuss the advantages and disadvantages of each approach.

An outline response is provided at the end of the chapter.

A standard experimental design (see Figure 1.2) includes a specification of who could be subjects or participants in the study and ensures that they are selected randomly and assigned at random to the conditions in the study.

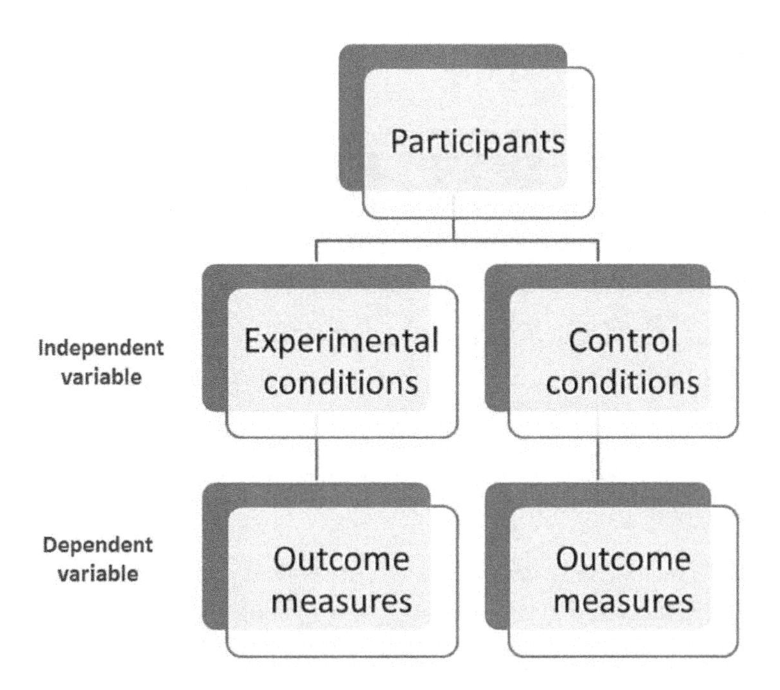

Figure 1.3: A standard experimental design

Randomised controlled trials (RCT)

Randomised controlled trials follow the principles of an experiment although, in most cases, it is impossible or undesirable to remove people from their normal lives to engage in a true experimental study. For instance, if we wanted to establish the impact of a new drug for depression, we would like to see the impact over time. We would aim to establish the differences in mood (dependent variable) over time between participants with a diagnosis of depression who have received the new drug in comparison with those who don't receive the drug (independent variable).

These days such a study would not just include one control group but also one that receives an established depression drug (market leader) as well as a placebo group. The mood of the participants would have to be significantly more improved in the experimental group (new drug) to justify putting the new drug on the market. I am sure you understand that it is very important that differences cannot be attributed to other variables. It is therefore necessary that participants are not aware of whether they are receiving the new drug, the market leader or the placebo. The impact might be affected by the expectations of the participants if they knew. This is called a blind study. It is also important that the experimenter's assistant involved in giving out the drugs or measuring mood is also not aware of which pills the participants have taken (double blind condition). It is not inconceivable that they would behave slightly differently if they knew in which group they were. They could, for instance, be slightly more enthusiastic with participants in the new drug group, which might affect the outcome. Of course, participants in such a study would most likely have very different life experiences in the course of the study, which is likely to cover several months. These differences are likely to affect the moods of the participants. Statistically it is expected that these variations may even out, as long as the group of participants is large enough. Studies such as in this example need to include thousands of participants before we can safely draw conclusions.

Activity 1.5 *Reflection*

Apply each of the research methods introduced in the above to study examples of issues in nursing. Start with naturalistic observation and work your way through in order.

An outline response is provided at the end of the chapter.

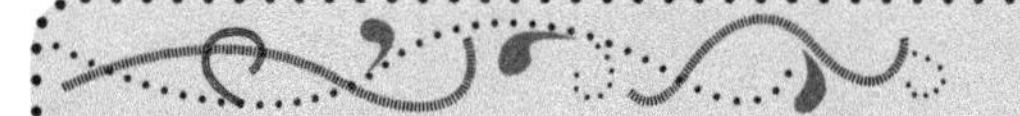

Chapter summary

- Psychology is included in nursing education because it is of practical use to nurses, it is relevant to health care, and it is prescribed by regulating bodies for nursing registration.
- Application of psychology should lead to better informed health care and a psychological mind-set supports more sophisticated approaches to nursing.

continued . . .

continued . . .

- Psychology is an essential element in the bio-psycho-social model and intertwined with health care and nursing.
- Psychological (and nursing) evidence is the result of empirical research of a quantitative and/or qualitative nature.
- Psychological research makes use of naturalistic observation, interviews, surveys, case studies, correlational studies, experiments, and randomised controlled trials.

Activities: brief outline answers

Activity 1.1: Reflection (see page 8)

This activity is intended to help you see how intertwined psychology is with health care and nursing. It is useful to explore the chapters related to the scenarios.

Scenario: Making contact

Each of the traditions of psychology suggests a different approach, but it is likely you will try out more than one. You might use empathy (humanistic), try to encourage the person (behavioural), or change the patient's mind-set (positive and/or cognitive psychology).

Scenario: Understanding the brain

Your interactions with doctors are based on mutual respect. Your understanding of the brain will help with this. This will also help you to understand your patients better.

Scenario: Development and learning

For example: very young children need to be rewarded; older children will understand what you would like to achieve; with older adults it is important not to take away their independent functioning.

Scenario: Nightshift

You need more REM sleep and find ways of getting it by ensuring you sleep longer.

Scenario: Under pressure

If you are still critically reflecting on what did not go right after your shift, you are highly conscientious. It is important to consider how to change your practice in response to this. Be aware that rational thinking can be affected by pressure.

Scenario: Group influence

Conformity and obedience play an important role. While they are needed in health care, they can cloud our independent judgement.

Scenario: Stress

You can tell yourself to remain positive, watch what you eat and keep your exercising going. If your voice matters in the hospital you might advocate increasing staffing and improving mood and attitude among staff.

Scenario: Illness as crisis

Sending the colleague away could increase the stress of the patient. Awareness of the patient's life will help you decide how to support him best.

Scenario: Person-centred versus task-oriented nursing

It is most likely you favoured nurse A but, when you are really busy, will you have time for Nurse A's approach? This is an important issue in contemporary health care.

Activity 1.2: Reflection (see page 9)

The answers are: a) biological; b) psychological; c) psychological and social; d) biological; e) biological and psychological; f) social and psychological. You may have found that all nursing activities that include personal contact include a psychological aspect.

Activity 1.3: Psychological mind-set (see page 10)

The outcome of the test is only meant for your reflection. It is not an official test instrument.

Activity 1.4: Quantitative versus qualitative research (see page 13)

The choice of approach depends on whether the hospital is more interested in satisfaction levels (quantitative) or what contributes to satisfaction (qualitative). On a practical level, answering the second question takes more time and it may not be feasible to ask all patients. In contrast, the first question might only take a minute and could be a standard part of the discharge procedure.

Concept Summary: lab, field and quasi-experiment (see page 15)

The advantage of the lab situation is that you can avoid disruptions, but not working with real patients is a major disadvantage. In the field experiment, real patients are an advantage, but it is impossible to control all that happens in a real hospital. The quasi-experiment may not show the clear dichotomy between the styles of Nurse A and Nurse B, but a more nuanced contrast; more realistic but, perhaps, findings will be less clear cut.

Activity 1.5: Reflection (see page 16)

Each of the approaches can be used in nursing studies. Hopefully, the exercise has given you an idea of how each method is relevant for different types of nursing questions

Further reading

Nolen-Hoeksema, S., Frederickson, B., Loftus, G. and Lutz, C. (2014) *Atkinson & Hilgard's Introduction to Psychology* (16th Ed.). Andover, Hampshire, UK; Cengage Learning.

Any general introduction to psychology can be read alongside this text for nurses, but this is a classic.

Weiten, W. (2008) *Psyk.Trek 3.1: A Multimedia Introduction to Psychology* (3rd Ed.). New York: Wadsworth.

This CD-ROM (or online access for Mac computers) provides perhaps the most accessible comprehensive introduction to psychology available.

Coon, D. and Mitterer, J. (2014) *Psychology: modules for active learning* (13th Ed.). Stamford, CT: Cengage Learning.

Dennis Coon is a master of introductory psychology who makes us all want to be psychologists.

Lilienfeld, S. O., Lynn, S. J., Ruscio, J. and Beyerstein, B. L. (2011) *50 great myths of popular psychology: Shattering widespread misconceptions about human behavior.* Chichester: Wiley-Blackwell.

Popular psychological perspectives include many myths. You will enjoy finding them debunked in convincing style.

Barley, E. (2016*) Health Psychology in Nursing Practice.* London: SAGE.

This short text will add to the understanding of health psychology and nursing in a most practical sense.

Useful websites

http://www.apa.org/action/

This is the public section of the American Psychological Association. You can use it to browse for psychological topics.

http://www.bbc.co.uk/programmes

BBC Horizon provides excellent programmes on the cusp of health and psychology.

http://www.open.edu/openlearn/health-sports-psychology/psychology/starting-psychology/content-section-0

The Open University in the UK has an open access section in which you can take modules on psychology.

http://list.ly/list/Gc-fun-psychology-related-youtube-videos

Psychology is well represented on YouTube. Use it but make sure you remain aware of what is serious and what is not. This is just fun!

https://www.youtube.com/watch?v=l49MzGZa_5M

This is a ten minute tutorial on Experimental Design. It covers lab., field and quasi-experiments.

Chapter 2
Understanding ourselves from various psychological perspectives

Chapter aims

After reading this chapter you will be able to:

- describe how psychology has developed as a field of study;
- discuss how the psychology of nursing developed in the twentieth century;
- discriminate between several schools of thought within psychology;
- apply the essential perspectives of the different schools of thought in psychology in nursing and health care.

This chapter outlines the history of psychology and psychology of/for nursing. We will look at psychological ideas from the late nineteenth and early twentieth centuries, from the eras of functionalism and structuralism, to the perspectives that are still influential today: psychodynamic psychology/psychoanalysis, behaviourism, cognitive, humanistic, social, evolutionary, positive, and biological psychology. With each different perspective we suggest how it is relevant in nursing and health care and provide opportunities to explore this.

The evolution of psychology

The history of psychology is, in essence, the history of how we understand the behaviour, actions and interactions of others and ourselves. Historical sources suggest that this fascination with understanding what shapes our actions and reactions goes back to ancient times. Even though, of course, limited evidence exists about this, archaeological and other historical evidence suggests a consistent human concern with knowing and understanding what it is to be human. The emergence of writing has provided lasting evidence of this interest and, indeed, significant efforts at understanding ourselves are to be found in early writings. Interestingly, religious works dominate, not only as sources that describe this understanding, but also because they contain teachings that influenced human thinking and behaviour in incredible ways. Sacred texts, such as the Bible and the Koran, were instrumental in codifying the required behaviour of these religions and were consistent with a growing moral development in humanity. Religious texts also ensured that 'believing' was an important feature of how we looked at the world and ourselves.

The rediscovery of the works of Greek philosophers, which were lost to many generations of Europeans until the Renaissance (fourteenth–seventeenth centuries), contributed greatly to the understanding of what we now call psychology. The focus on 'knowing' rather than 'believing', as expressed by the likes of Plato, Aristotle and Socrates, inspired many a European scholar. The Age of Enlightenment saw this principle extend into wider society and, increasingly, West European philosophers asked and attempted to answer complex questions about the human condition. The invention of print facilitated the free flow of ideas and the dialectic process of thesis and antithesis by which philosophy developed. The relationship between body and soul was a topic of hot debate. The nature<>nurture debate is another good example. Much of how we think about ourselves has been a matter of long-lasting polemics and disagreements. In particular, the intricacy and versatility of nineteenth-century European debates on thinking, consciousness, evolution, psychophysics and related topics formed a rich breeding ground for the next step: the call for empirical research on ourselves. In most introductory psychology texts this period is considered the time when psychology as we know it today was established.

The emergence of empirical psychology in the nineteenth century

The nineteenth century was an exciting time in the history of science. It is characterised by the development of technology, industrialisation, colonialism, education, and a gradual process of secularisation of science in the Western world. All of these elements facilitated an emphasis on rationality and empirical research. It was almost inevitable that this would also involve the study of human thinking and perception. It is no coincidence that much of the development in the early nineteenth century took place in Germany. A powerhouse of science and philosophy had become interested in testing not just physics theories but also aspects of our own functioning. In particular, Theodore Fechner (1801–1887) and Ernst-Heinrich Weber (1795–1878) who introduced **psychophysics** – often seen as an early form of psychology – paved the way. The psychophysicists ambitiously applied laws of physics to study the human experience in the belief that 'the mental and the material are two coequal aspects of the same underlying reality' (Lowry, 1971, p. 93). Wilhelm Wundt's (1832–1920) elaborate efforts to establish an empirical psychology followed in their footsteps. His founding of the first psychological lab in the world in Leipzig in 1879 is often seen as a landmark. He and his collaborators executed strictly controlled laboratory experiments in an attempt to establish the structure of conscious experience. His subjects were, for instance, strapped into contraptions that isolated different muscle groups and then asked to give an account of this experience. In another experiment they were asked to reflect on simple thought processes while they took place. In English this was referred to as 'introspection'. Wundt's English student Edward Titchener (1867–1927) introduced (and adapted) his work in Britain and America. Their early efforts are usually indicated as **structuralism** because of its emphasis on the structure of the conscious experience.

Around the same time the balance of influence in the world of science was starting to shift to the USA. While the structuralists certainly had an impact across the Atlantic, a different perspective also gained ground, in particular through the efforts of the American William James (1842–1910). His publication of *The Principles of Psychology* (James, 1890) indicates a shift towards a pragmatic perspective of psychology. Heavily influenced by Darwin's evolution theory he emphasised the need to explore everyday psychological phenomena such as the function of emotions, consciousness, habits and instincts. This approach to psychology, which was shared by many other American psychologists of that era, was often referred to as **functionalism**.

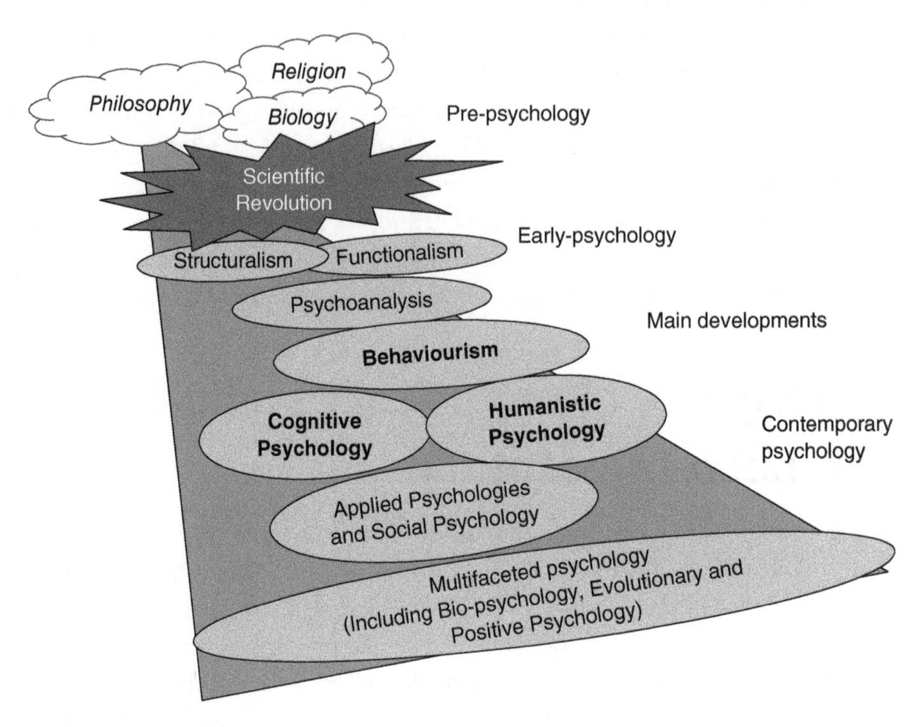

Figure 2.1: How psychology evolved

In talking about Charles Darwin (1809–1882), and other theorists on **evolutionary theory** who did not become as popular (for example, Wallace 1823–1913), we need to emphasise the importance of the publication of *On the Origin of Species* (Darwin, 1859). Its impact on the emergence of psychology is perhaps best described as one of kicking open the door unlocked by the psychophysicists for the empirical method in the study of humans. Evolutionary theory suggested that humans were not different from animals, in the sense that we had evolved from other species. At the time Darwin was frequently attacked and mocked for what were considered very radical ideas.

Nonetheless, the thought took hold among fellow scientists that if we could study animals empirically, then this approach could also be used to study humans. The familial relationship between humans and all mammals was later also used as an argument by the behaviourists (see below) for animal research to make inferences about human learning.

In the same period we also see a significant change in perspective on mental illness and treatment that initiated the development of **psychiatry** as a field. By 1800 the thought that people with mental health problems were possessed by the devil or engaged in witchcraft had more or less been abandoned. Nonetheless, the special institutions set up to care for (but mainly control) them, evolved only slowly. Lack of insight in psychopathology and treatment effectiveness played an important role (Eling *et al.*, 2013). Nonetheless, such institutions became a place where changing perspectives on psychopathology developed. In particular the French institute

La Salpêtrière played a pivotal role in this process. Philippe Pinel (1745–1826) has gone down in history as the person who started the process of (literally) freeing psychiatric patients of their chains. While a more humane approach to care developed, causes for psychopathology were increasingly equated with neuropathology, in particular in brain tissue. Although this was a sign of things to come, there were also forces that suggested an independent psychiatry separate from neurology. In particular, Kraepelin's (1856–1926) systematic development of diagnostics and prognosis based on research seemed to give psychiatry a focus in its own right, without a need for a neurological underpinning. By the end of the nineteenth century he had developed a diagnostic system that later became the basis for the development of the Diagnostic and Statistical Manual of Mental Disorders (DSM).

Around the same time, both in the USA and Europe, the interest in psychopathology in everyday life became a hot issue. The work of Sigmund Freud (1856–1939) is a good example of this. Starting out as a family doctor in Vienna he became interested in the hidden psychological causes of the physical issues his patients presented with. He was perhaps the most influential of exponents of this development and his theoretical work on the subconscious, psychosexual development, dreams, and the development of **psychoanalysis** as a form of treatment through 'talk', revolutionised both psychiatry and psychology. After structuralism and functionalism this is generally seen as the third force that shaped psychology around the turn of the century in 1900. Its impact is still with us.

Concept summary: Psychodynamic/psychoanalytic perspective – discovering what is hidden in us (unconscious)

A lot of human mental activity is hidden in our subconscious and we are not aware of much of its machinations. To understand ourselves we should aim to unlock these mysteries, which come to the surface in our dreams and fantasies and make use of intricate symbols. Much of our personal development has its roots in our early childhood.

Applications to nursing and health care:

- nurses may have essential unconscious motivations for their work;
- unconscious mental health issues may contribute to physical health problems;
- nurses should consider exploring unconscious psychological factors that might block recovery in patients or clients.

Psychology in the twentieth and twenty-first centuries

The development of psychology in general is best understood as a series of lengthy debates among contrasting and conflicting perspectives. This is particularly true for the twentieth century. Psychology has only recently come to some form of synthesis. We will attempt to highlight the essence of the developments in a nutshell. The early twentieth century saw the emergence of what quickly became a fight for dominance, or perhaps 'ownership' is a better word, within the budding field of psychology. Although the structuralist and functionalist perspectives had advocated a psychology of empirical research, it was a major problem that doing research on what goes on in our heads in an objective manner was (and is) very difficult. While Freud and other psychoanalysts worked tirelessly on the development of theories of the conscious and subconscious mind using case studies, a new movement emerged that considered this a dead end street for a scientific psychology.

This approach was referred to as **behaviourism.** Early behaviourists claimed that psychologists should only study observable behaviour and how it varies in response to stimuli from the environment. While they did not deny that humans think and have emotions, behaviourists argued that because we cannot observe these phenomena reliably, let alone measure them, these should be placed outside of the field of study. They considered all mental activity as inaccessible to scientific study: as if taking place in a 'black box'. Ivan Pavlov's (1849–1936) studies of salivation in dogs in 1904, which led to the discovery of an important principle of learning (classical conditioning – see Chapter 4), are often considered to have provided the impetus for this development.

The American John Watson (1878–1958), who was involved in similar research at that time, proceeded to test the principles of conditioning in humans (the infamous Little Albert Study – see Chapter 4) (Watson and Rayner, 1920). His work and that of many others, including B.F. Skinner (1904–1990), established the development of the behaviourist perspective as the dominant approach within the field. Skinner's research, mainly using rats and other animals, helped develop theories of how reward and punishment affect behaviour. He called this 'operant conditioning' (see Chapter 6). Skinner was a prolific author and, arguably, one of the most influential psychologists of the twentieth century. Interestingly, he also applied his principles in a utopian novel (Skinner and Hayes, 1976) and a popular text with a persuasive argument suggesting that the world works entirely based on behaviourist principles (Skinner, 1972).

Concept summary: Behavioural perspective – understanding learning and behaviour in response to the environment

Most relevant about human beings is not that we think or feel, but what we do. Overt behaviour and what controls it should be the core of the psychological enterprise. We are all subject to Thorndike's law of effect, which states that behaviours that lead to desirable consequences are more likely to be repeated, while behaviours that lead to undesirable consequences are less likely to reoccur. How we learn is an important focal point of behaviourist research.

Applications to nursing and health care:

- how nursing skills are learned should be a topic of study;
- effective nursing makes use of encouragement (reward) and discouragement (punishment) in interactions with patients/clients/service users;
- unlearning unhealthy behaviours and learning healthy ones is key to health promotion.

The reaction to behaviourism came in several waves. Firstly, the psychoanalytical movement had not subsided. Its theoretical perspectives found a broad following and there was a growing interest in its method of treating people with mental health problems. Freud, but also Jung, Adler and others, had ambitiously worked on developing comprehensive theories that were conspicuously delving into mental functioning, conscious and subconscious. By ignoring the behaviourists' call to leave mental activity alone, psychoanalytic theory maintained the status of an inspiring alternative. Secondly, the **Gestalt psychology** movement, which emerged at around the same time as behaviourism, was still looking for a way of studying the 'mind'. Using the principle of totality, they advocated a psychology that looked at the 'whole' as other than separate aspects of experiences (Koffka, 1921) and would seek scientific evidence not through lab experiments but through real-life experiments in daily reality. This inspired the **humanistic perspective**, which came to the forefront a few decades later. The humanists dismissed animal research as not very useful in shedding light on specifically human issues. Also, while critical of the psychoanalytical emphasis on what is hidden and what is wrong with people, humanists set out a new agenda of promoting a more positive perspective on human functioning rooted in the winning ideology of the 'American Dream' (democracy, human rights, freedom, opportunities for all, equality, capitalism). It is no coincidence that the outcome of the Second World War contributed considerably to its support in the 'Free West'. The promotion of democracy coincided with the assumption that people have the power to make real choices about their lives, instead of being simply the product of their genetic predispositions and environmental influences. The existence of 'free will' and the idea of the independent 'self' as central to psychology became dominant features in the debates around understanding ourselves. Carl Rogers (1902–1987) and Abraham Maslow (1909–1970) are among the most influential humanists. Most importantly, Rogers developed the principles and method of 'client-centred therapy', the foundation of 'person-centred care' (see Chapter 10) and Maslow suggested a 'hierarchy of needs' (see Chapter 8) to which contemporary psychology and nursing texts still refer.

Concept summary: Humanist perspective – understanding and developing what is typically human in us

We cannot study psychology without focussing on the specifically human experience. It is essential to study how we see and experience ourselves and how we are motivated to give meaning to our lives. Humans have dignity and purpose because we have free will to shape our lives. This is the *origin of person-centred care.* Skills like good listening, demonstrating empathy, and providing emotional support, have been developed and described within the humanistic perspective.

Applications to nursing and health care:

- person-centred care and how it is practised is essential in health care today;
- a strong therapeutic relationship in health care is based on humanistic principles;
- we need to understand what motivates care giver and care receiver.

A third wave – **cognitive psychology** – was a matter of science overtaking the principle of the 'black box'. With Noam Chomsky's (1928–) unrelenting criticism of Skinner as the catalyst, the 'cognitive revolution' really took flight with the invention of the computer. Those psychologists still interested in studying cognition now had a means of modelling human thinking. They developed 'information processing' models as the basis for research on humans (memory, decision making, problem solving, risk assessment, etc.). The computer helped us see that the 'black box' was perhaps not so black anymore. Cognitive psychologists such as Gardner argued that if we allowed computers to think then surely we should allow humans to do so (Gardner, 2008)! Of course, more recent developments allow us an increasingly detailed peek into the brain through EEG, PET and fMRI, which has put the study of thinking fully back on the agenda.

Concept summary: Cognitive perspective – understanding how we think

We all experience our world and ourselves in profoundly different ways, because we think differently. Hence we need to study thinking and related mental efforts (cognition) as part of a meaningful psychology. Cognitive psychologists are very interested in how irrational and negative thinking can be transformed into rational and positive thinking.

Applications to nursing and health care:

- what nurses think is important for the quality of their care;
- nurses often affect the thinking and attitudes of people in their care;
- our thinking about health and illness affects health behaviours.

So, while the Gestalt psychologists and humanists developed theories of higher order functioning and new and revolutionary approaches to psychotherapy, the psychoanalysts continued their quest under the new name of psychodynamic psychology, and cognitive psychologists came out of the closet. In the 1960s and 70s the interest in psychotherapy reached almost epidemic forms under well-to-do intellectuals and it should not surprise us that, by that time, each of the schools of thought boasted a psychotherapy branch. In the meantime, applied psychological research started to take over from the strict behaviourist perspective. Between the 1920s and the 1970s we see the true birth of a diverse psychology with an ever-growing empirical ethos on the one hand and the energy to impact society and the lives of individuals, including their mental health, on the other hand. We see the emergence of psychometric psychology, developmental or life span psychology (Piaget), social psychology (Lewin, Milgram, Asch), personality and differential psychology (Allport, Eysenck), and the social cognitive perspective (Bandura).

Perhaps among the most influential of these fields is **social psychology**. While on the one hand an applied field, it has become increasingly evident that the social psychological perspective, which approaches the study of psychology always from the perspective of the social context, makes a unique contribution to our understanding of psychology in general. Specifically, we have to thank ingenious and bold researchers such as Leon Festinger (1991–1989), Stanley Milgram (1933–1984) and Philip Zimbardo (1933–) for social psychological experiments that have significantly altered the way in which we understand the impact of others on us. It is safe to say that experiments on cognitive dissonance, obedience, conformity and role behaviour have shocked the world by demonstrating how prepared we are to do things against our better judgement when under social pressure. In the wake of the Second World War, our understanding of the darker side of humanity has been advanced rapidly by social psychology. Many social psychological studies that took place between 1950 and 1980 epitomise the empirical drive within the history of psychology and are therefore at the core of its development. We'll come back to this in Chapter 7.

Concept summary: Social psychology – understanding social interactions and social influence

We are social animals. Our behaviour and our thinking is affected by others and by the social situations in which we find ourselves. We often underestimate this. The power of situations is strong enough to make us think and do things that go against our personal principles.

Applications to nursing and health care:

- nurses and patients are affected by the strong impact of health-care organisations;
- there is a need to assess social factors that affect health and illness;
- the impact of social situations can cloud our judgement in health care.

Activity 2.1 — *The top ten psychologists in the twentieth century (Dittman, 2002)*

These psychologists are the most cited overall, most cited in introductory psychology texts and most nominated by experts in the twentieth century. Look up these names online and write a short paragraph about each author. This will add to the depth of your understanding of psychology.

1. B.F. Skinner
2. Jean Piaget
3. Sigmund Freud
4. Albert Bandura
5. Leon Festinger
6. Carl R. Rogers
7. Stanley Schachter
8. Neal E. Miller
9. Edward Thorndike
10. A.H. Maslow

An outline answer is provided at the end of the chapter.

Most recent developments

While some of the proponents of the initial schools of thought in psychology claimed that their perspective could be used as a basis for studying all aspects of the field, the reality today is that many psychologists see themselves as eclectic or influenced by more than one approach. In the 1980s it was still common for psychologists to distinguish themselves from others by mentioning their allegiance to one of these schools of thought. Today psychologists who still identify as behaviourist, psychodynamic or humanistic psychologists are considered to be living in the past! Contemporary psychologists are identified generally according to their particular area of study, or even the topic within this area.

Several specific fields such as educational psychology, cultural psychology, occupational psychology, organisational psychology, forensic psychology, cognitive neuroscience, and indeed health psychology have emerged and thrived in the second half of the twentieth century. Each of these fields has a focus on a particular area of human functioning and is, to a large extent, a response to demands in society to address specific issues. This development is part of an increasing level of professionalisation in an ever-expanding field. While, of course, this is a success story, we need to be aware that the exponential growth and increasing specialisation within psychology have come at a price. Today very few psychologists still possess the broad generalist knowledge to interrelate the different areas. This threatens to fragment the field. Surprisingly, it is often the popular psychological publications, in their efforts to translate psychological principles for the general public, which succeed in connecting elements in a field that had grown apart.

Activity 2.2 ***Popular psychology***

Here is our top ten of popular psychology books. We've selected a variety of books and have probably omitted important ones. Perhaps you have your own favourites. You can look up these books online and read reviews. Try to establish the core ideas in each book.

1. Daniel Kahneman – *Thinking fast and slow*
2. Richard Dawkins – *The selfish gene*
3. Daniel Goleman – *Emotional intelligence*
4. Ellen Langer – *Mindfulness*
5. Carol Tavris and Elliot Aronson – *Mistakes were made but not by me*
6. Oliver Sachs – *The man who mistook his wife for his hat*
7. Malcolm Gladwell – *Blink*
8. Mihaly Csikszentmihalyi – *Flow: the psychology of optimal experience*
9. Tony Buzan – *Use your memory*
10. David Coleman – *The thriving family*

It is fortunate that new overarching perspectives on the field as a whole have also reminded us that beyond all the specialisation there are fundamental nuts to be cracked. **Bio-psychology** is of particular importance because it advocates a perspective that is closely related to biology. While it is some time since we moved on from the dualistic view that mind and body are separate entities, the integrated study has been held back by the complexity of the relationship between biology and psychology. However, from the 1990s onwards, we see several developments that tread on this pathway. **Cognitive neuroscience** is a good example. Major advances in this area have taken place in the last 20 years, with a rosy future in sight. Health psychology and behavioural medicine each follow the same integrative perspective, as do specific fields like psycho-immunology, psycho-oncology, and psycho-neuro-endocrinology and behavioural genetics. Developments within clinical psychology and psychiatry also emphasise the exploration of this relationship. While we should not consider the scope of bio-psychology as new, it is important to highlight that its prominence has changed how psychology is practised and perceived.

Concept summary: Bio-psychology – integrating psychology and biology

This perspective looks at how the biological functions and structure of the human system interact with psychological manifestations. The core principle is that human behaviour, emotions and cognition cannot be fully understood without integrating the biological and psychological aspect.

Applications to nursing and health care:

- biological and psychological knowledge needs to be used in tandem by nurses and doctors;
- biological and psychological factors interact in health, mental health, illness, disability and ageing;
- patients need to be educated on how biological factors affect them psychologically and vice versa.

A similar multi-disciplinary effort to expand psychology emerged in the form of **evolutionary psychology**. Rooted in evolutionary theory and using evidence from such diverse fields as behavioural genetics, biology, archaeology, sociology, history and anthropology, its main focus is on studying our behaviour and mental and social functioning as based on adaptations that have evolved over many generations within our species and, before that, in other mammals. Not entirely unlike the functionalists, evolutionary psychologists tend to ask the questions 'what is the original function of behaviours, emotions and cognition?' and 'how did these manifestations help us survive and reproduce?' (Buss, 1999). With more and more fundamental evidence about our distant past emerging, we are better able than ever before to map out what happened in the period of human history when the survival pressure was particularly high: the long period in which we lived a nomadic existence as hunter-gatherers. It is thought that at one point we were close to extinction. It is of particular interest to study which emerging features (adaptations) helped us survive during this time, because these may be the same qualities that make us so resilient today. Evolutionary psychologists are also interested in how the ancient 'hunter-gatherer' in us deals with the profoundly different circumstances in which we live our lives today.

Concept summary: Evolutionary psychology – understanding the 'hunter-gatherer' within us

How we behave, think, feel and interact with others is, to a large extent, rooted in how we developed as a species. We need to study ourselves with this in mind and identify how survival and reproduction have shaped our species physically and psychologically. We should also ask whether seemingly maladaptive behaviours in today's world may have been adaptive in the era in which they developed, when we still lived as hunter-gatherers. Some of these tendencies are hard to override.

Applications to nursing and health care:

- many people find it hard to control what they eat because of evolutionary 'programming';
- nurses need to overrule seemingly innate bias against people who are 'different';
- many intuitive and subconscious responses in health care have their roots in the 'hunter-gatherer in us'.

At about the same time **positive psychology** (Seligman and Csikszentmihalyi, 2000) was launched as a response to all overly problem-focused approaches within the field. Seligman made a case for the fact that not enough was done to study the positive, adaptive and creative aspects of the human experience and that there was a need to remedy this. Evolutionary and positive psychology have motivated us to ask new questions, take a fresh perspective on old issues, and propose new hypotheses and solutions. These exciting developments have rejuvenated psychology and attest to the fact that the mission of psychology is continuing with renewed inspiration in the twenty-first century.

Concept summary: Positive psychology – using psychology in positive ways

Too much of psychology is focused on our weaknesses. We should study our strengths more in order to harness what can assist us in being effective, healthy and happy in this world. Psychology should progress in its efforts to have a positive impact on humanity.

Applications to nursing, patients and health care:

- use of optimism in nursing care;
- health benefits of positive thinking;
- develop ways of learning to become more positive.

Table 2.1: Core focus of main contemporary perspectives on psychology

Perspective on psychology (and main theorists)	Core focus
Psychoanalysis or Psychodynamic psychology (Freud, Jung)	Discovering what is hidden in us (unconscious)
Behaviourism (Pavlov, Watson, Skinner)	Understanding how we learn and behave in response to the environment
Humanism (Rogers, Maslow)	Understanding and developing what is typically human in us
Cognitive psychology (Chomsky, Beck, Ellis)	Understanding how we think
Social psychology (Festinger, Milgram, Asch, Zimbardo)	Understanding social interactions and social influence
Biological psychology (Lorenz, Tinbergen, Penfield)	Integrating psychology and biology in understanding human behaviour, emotions and cognition
Evolutionary psychology (Darwin, Buss, Tooby and Cosmides)	Understanding the 'hunter-gatherer' within us
Positive psychology (Seligman)	Developing and using psychology in positive ways

The big picture

It would appear that the overall history of what we describe today as psychology seems to highlight a shifting interest over time with, initially, a strong focus on the soul, then consciousness, then behaviour, then emotion and cognition, and then today all manifestations of the human experience tied in with biological and social aspects. The industrial revolution and colonialism, while generating immense wealth in the Western world, has advanced our understanding of ourselves, when we thrive and when we suffer. This has propelled the interest in psychology forward. The intense turmoil in the last century with several incisive wars and the ideological battle between capitalism and communism has also significantly impacted the field. Urbanisation, globalisation, the information boom, the Internet, concerns about the environment, global warming, immigration and significant political shifts have since continued to alter our world and with it the focus of psychology and its applications. While much of the development of psychology so far has taken place in the Western world there are signs that this is changing. This is important because a mature psychology should be applicable to different cultures and incorporate different ways of living. Undoubtedly, future developments will continue to change the field because what is the point of psychology if it does not address current life and issues?

The development of a psychology for/of nursing

Perhaps the earliest textbook of psychology for nurses (Burr, 1906) was meant for psychiatric nurses and presented mainly psychoanalytical theory. Soon after, several comprehensive texts reflective of the psychology of that time started to appear in the USA (Muse, 1925). The American Committee on Education of the National League of Nursing Education had started recommending that psychology be included in nursing education. They specifically emphasised that psychological content should consist of: a stating of principles of human conduct; how to deal effectively with patients; development of principles of dealing wisely with patients and colleagues; helping the student to achieve self-mastery in work and private life; and providing a basis for further study in psychiatry and ethics (Higgins, 1921). The benefits of psychology were generally introduced with great enthusiasm (de Vries and Timmins, 2012) and psychology was hailed as an important contribution to the understanding of patients' minds and the professionalism of nurses (Forbes, 1919). The fast development of psychology at that time is reflected in significantly altered new editions (such as Muse (1934)) appearing within only a few years of its first publication. The mandated introduction of psychology as part of the nursing curriculum in Britain and Ireland in the 1950s boosts the introduction of British psychology texts for nurses such as Odlum (1952), which also appears in regularly updated editions for a number of decades. More recent texts have by now also appeared in several editions (Walker *et al.*, 2012; Gross and Kinnison, 2014; Rana and Upton, 2013). The significant differences in these texts reflect that the application of psychology to nursing has not crystallised fully and there is still debate about which aspects of psychology are most relevant for nurses.

It is evident that, of the schools of thought in psychology, humanistic psychology has had the most significant impact in guiding contemporary principles of care provision. Specifically the introduction of the principles of **person-centred** care can be traced back to Carl Rogers' (1902–1987) work on client-centred therapy (Rogers, 1951). Along with other exponents of humanism, his work is well integrated in the principles taught in nursing education today. Furthermore, principles of behaviourism and cognitive psychology have been absorbed in health promotion and behavioural change, communication skills, and other activities in which nurses are involved. In addition to this, the emergence of health psychology has provided impetus for the introduction of a new evidence base for nursing and health care. We would, however, argue that many fundamental aspects of psychology have relevance for nurses and that therefore it is useful for nurses to acquire a fundamental understanding of psychology in general. We need to keep in mind that the relevance of psychology *for* nurses goes beyond a psychology *of* nursing. The former would include an effort towards a broad application of psychology to benefit nursing and health care, starting out from psychology. The latter would originate within nursing and aims to investigate which aspects of psychology are useful to clarify principles of nursing and issues of relevance to nurses. This book ventures into both approaches.

Just like with psychology in general, it is developments in the world that shape the field of psychology of/for nursing. In our case, the field is focused by developments in global health, political perspectives on where health care should be situated (in hospitals or in the community?), the role of health promotion, and issues like nutrition, epidemics, poverty, and health-care scandals. Where possible this book will relate to these developments. For the moment, nothing stands in your way to pick and choose which elements and perspectives within psychology inspire you most. Just like in Chapter 1, we have provided you with several opportunities to relate psychology with nursing in theory and in practice. We'll round off with a final chance to check that you can make sense of the different perspectives in psychology and recognise how they apply in nursing (see Activity 2.3).

Activity 2.3 — *The magnificent eight*

Table 2.1 (see p 31) describes eight different perspectives on psychology. Each one of them has been applied to nursing. Can you figure out which psychological perspective is at the basis of how these nurses express their views on care?

(a) .... : I try to make people feel appreciated and understood, and maintain a sense of purpose in life.

(b) .... : I will do my best to encourage positive health behaviours and ensure that new skills to enhance health are well learned.

(c) .... : I am always interested in what is going on subconsciously in the patients. This contains important clues as to their real needs.

(d) .... : Winning over my patients into thinking in rational ways about their illness is essential to how I approach their care.

Psychology ???

(e) .... : Optimism and resilience are the qualities I seek to promote. I also emphasise ability over disability.

(f) .... : I mostly focus on how physical issues, behaviour and mental aspects of the patient's health connect.

(g) .... : I often assume that the way in which a patient responds intuitively to their situation has a grounding in the ability to survive.

(h) .... : Hospitals and other health-care facilities constitute very powerful environments with an important impact on patients and staff.

When you've completed the task, please discuss and add to the content of each box in a way that makes sense to you.

An outline answer is provided at the end of the chapter.

Chapter summary

- Psychology is not a recent development but, as a field of empirical research, it only emerged in the second half of the nineteenth century.

continued . . .

continued . . .

- Different schools of thought have been involved in struggles for dominance and vociferous debate within the field, which has gradually led to the acceptance that each perspective contributes in a meaningful way.
- There is no crystallised psychology of nursing at present. Different psychological texts for nurses use a wide variety of approaches.
- In nursing and health care the humanistic perspective dominates, but behavioural, cognitive, social and positive psychology each contribute considerably to the understanding of issues and interventions.
- A well-informed nurse will make use of several of these psychological perspectives.

Activities: brief outline answers

Activity 2.1: Top ten psychologists (see page 27)

There are many more important psychologists. We already see that new names have emerged. Psychology has been dominated by men but that is changing. Look up, for example, Elizabeth Loftus, Ellen Langer, Karen Horney and Margaret Washburn.

Activity 2.2: Popular psychology (see page 28)

Each of these books has changed the minds of the public on important psychological phenomena.

Activity 2.3: The magnificent eight (see page 33)

The answers are: a) Humanism; b) Behaviourism; c) Psychodynamic/Psychoanalysis; d) Cognitive; e) Positive psychology; f) Biopsychology; g) Evolutionary psychology; h) Social psychology.

Further reading

Schultz, D. and Schultz, S. (2015) *A history of modern psychology* (11th Ed). Boston: Cengage Learning.

There are several good overviews of the history of psychology. This text is lively and accessible. You may find access online to read bits and pieces.

Hock, R. R. (2013) *Forty studies that changed psychology* (7th Ed). Pearson Higher Education.

Psychology is best understood by learning about research studies. This provides a good overview.

Reber, A. S., Allen, R. and Reber, E. S. (2009) *Penguin dictionary of psychology* (4th ed). London: Penguin Press.

If you are quicker with a reference book than with Wikipedia on-line, this would be a good choice.

Harari, Yuval Noah (2014) *Sapiens: a brief history of humankind.* New York: Random House.

Lucid and surprising perspective on the history of our species with psychological implications.

Useful websites

http://www.apa.org/monitor/julaug02/eminent.aspx

This list of the most influential psychologists in the twentieth century has been cited many times.

http://www.learner.org/series/discoveringpsychology/history/history_flash.html

Annenberg Learner provides several important features to help students and teachers to enrich psychology modules.

https://www.youtube.com/watch?v=CsxKcY94EB4

When you look up 'History of Psychology' in YouTube you will most likely stumble on videos or slide presentations that provide an overview in 5-10 minutes. Well worth the time!

Chapter 3
The core of our functioning and how we make sense of our world

Chapter aims

After reading this chapter you will be able to:

- outline the psychological implications of the function and structure of the nervous and endocrine systems and, more specifically, how our activities, thinking and emotions are generated by our nervous system and, in particular, by the brain;
- describe the ways in which the organisation and functioning of our nervous system (and specifically our brain) may facilitate as well as complicate our psychological functioning;
- discuss your understanding of the brain and nervous system and related matters in a multi-disciplinary team;
- explain how the human system receives information from the outside world and its own body (sensation) and makes sense of this information (perception);
- understand how we are prone to make mistakes and miscalculations in how we perceive our environment.

In this chapter we will focus on our core psychological functions, how the human system gathers and processes information from the outside world and from within itself, and how we make sense of that information. The complexity of these processes in humans surpasses all other organisms on this planet and generates a unique ability to survive, reproduce, learn and adapt in constantly changing circumstances. Nurses learn about the nervous, endocrine and sensory systems in biology classes, but they need to relate this knowledge to understanding themselves and their patients psychologically. The chapter also focuses on sensation and perception: vision, hearing and the other senses. As a matter of safety, we include perceptual principles and illusions, because our senses and perceptual faculties may deceive us.

The human system and its main functions

A child gets a new toy, turns it upside down, takes a good look, and asks 'what is it supposed to do?' This is essentially the same question an engineer would ask first when designing machinery, a system, equipment or a building: What does it need to do? What is it for? What is its function? When we look at ourselves we often get overwhelmed by the complexity of biological structures, psychological mechanisms and social interactions. As a result we often fail to make sense of the core functions of the human system. We need to turn things around and, just like the child and the engineer, start by establishing what humans are supposed to be able to do. Once we've answered this question we will be much better placed to make sense of it all.

So what are humans supposed to do? At its most primary level the answer is simple: survive and reproduce (see Figure 3.1). Other functions should be seen as essentially leading towards these two primary aims. Seeking access to nutrients (sustenance) and protecting ourselves are secondary aims to achieve survival, while sex and care for offspring are secondary aims towards reproduction. At a third level we can identify behavioural tendencies, motivations and emotions that spur us to remain engaged in these activities. Overarching functions such as movement, sensation and perception, learning, development, play, consciousness, memory, thinking, competition, collaboration, social support, etc. serve more than one purpose. If we want to make sense of ourselves we need to make the connection between how the system is biologically organised and how psychological functions of our system are facilitated.

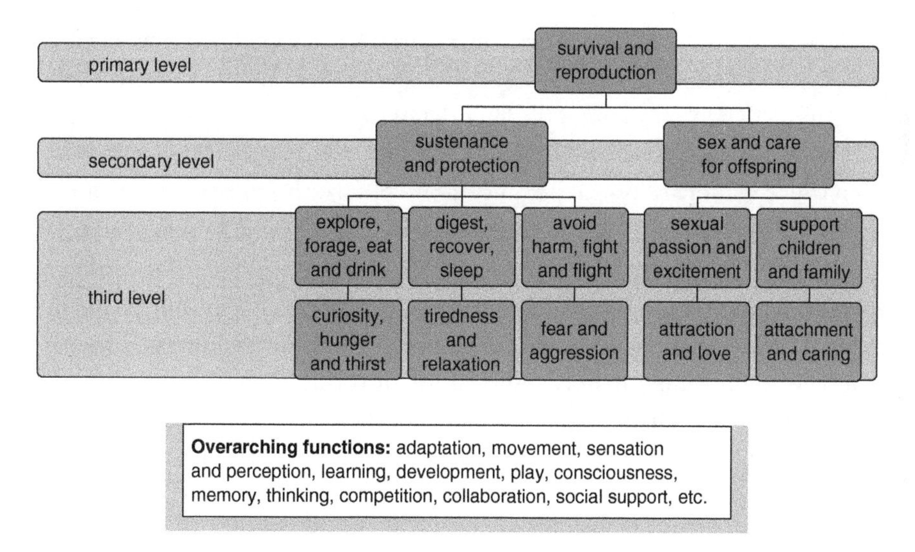

Figure 3.1: The main functions in human life

Survival and reproduction are essential functions that both have biological and psychological aspects. The immediate survival of the system relies on the organisation of cells in systems with specific functions. Each of these systems is vital. If your circulatory system stops working, oxygen will no longer reach the cells and death is imminent. If the digestive system stops, nutrients will cease to be transported to the cells, which will also mean that the end is in sight. With different degrees of urgency, the same point can be made for all other systems. Psychological aspects such as hunger, thirst and the strong emotions we experience when we are in danger or found in need, play an essential role in motivating survival behaviour.

For reproduction the same argument can be made. Hormonal and fertility aspects (biology) enable reproduction, while emotions, motivation and behaviour (psychology) are essential to finding a partner and mate. Many psychological aspects are as much impacted by our genes as biological ones. There is significant evidence to suggest that personality, intelligence, resilience, and mental health have a genetic basis (Plomin *et al.*, 2013). Also, temperamental factors such as shyness and openness to experience are inherited through our genes (Kagan *et al.*, 1988). Dawkins (2006) goes as far as to suggest that our DNA is essentially pulling the strings in the background for all major psychological tendencies and activities (see the Concept summary below).

Concept summary: My genes made me do it!

In *The Selfish Gene* Richard Dawkins presents the case for the relationship between our genes and us as one of slavery. Our genes build us with the only objective of creating a host that secures their eternal life from generation to generation (Dawkins, 2006). Dawkins posits that 'the fundamental unit of selection, and therefore of self-interest, is not the species, nor the group, nor even, strictly the individual. It is the gene, the unit of heredity' (Dawkins, 2006, p. 11). In his view we are essentially instruments in the service of genes that have programmed us to perform activities to aid survival and reproduction. This explains why people flee without thinking when overpowered by fear in life-threatening situations, or why we become helpless when enchanted by the attractiveness of a potential partner. The strength of these urges is genetically programmed in us and often overrules reason and rationality. If Dawkins' ideas had not been so contrary to our sense of control of our lives, then you would hear this excuse much more often: 'My genes made me do it!'

As regards nursing, it is important to consider how nursing care fits in with the main functions of human life. It would make sense to think that nurses draw on an inherited preparedness to support and care that, while innately reserved for offspring, family and community, can be extended to patients and clients once an attachment (therapeutic relationship) is formed. Furthermore, your own sustenance (work–pay–food) and protection are at stake and motivate your efforts to do well and work in safe ways.

Activity 3.1 — *Reflection*

Reflect on how the functions in Figure 3.1 affect you in your role as a nurse. How do you foster a personal connection with patients to trigger your preparedness to provide care and support? What do you do to protect yourself from harm? How do you ensure you get enough rest and sleep?

The nervous system and its psychological functions

The **nervous system** is built up of connecting neurons that process information. It comprises a central part, the central nervous system, which includes brain and spinal cord, and the peripheral nervous system, which consists of the somatic, sympathetic and parasympathetic nervous systems (see Figure 3.2). Each of these systems is involved in the coordination of psychological functions. We will highlight these as we address each system.

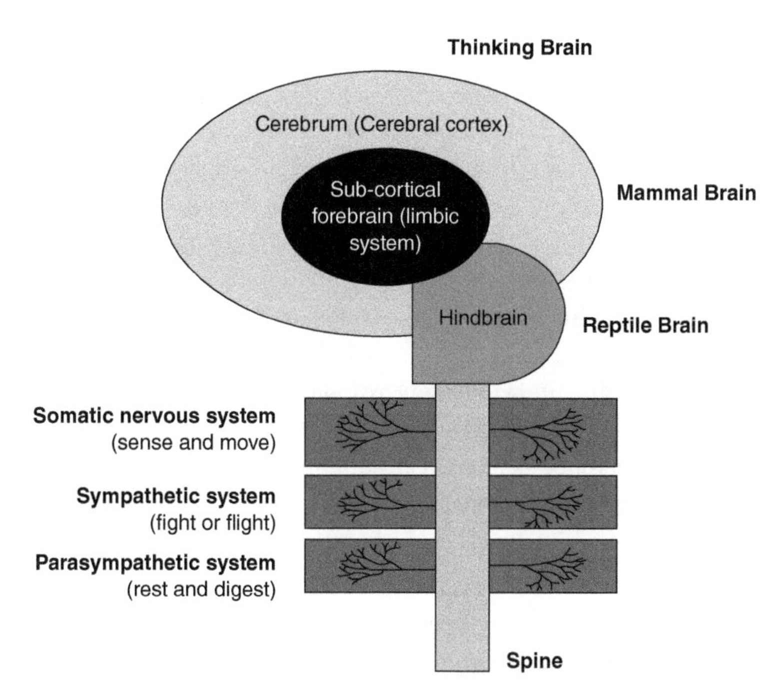

Figure 3.2: Diagram of the nervous system

Let us discuss the peripheral system first.

The peripheral nervous system (PNS)

The PNS consists of three separate sections. Within these three sections, each with a different function, incoming (afferent) and outgoing (efferent) signals make use of separate neural pathways. Overall, the three sections represent the three functions under the 'sustenance and protection' section of the model of the main functions of the human system (Figure 3.1).

Within the PNS, the **somatic nervous system** connects the muscles and senses with the spine and the brain. Thus it facilitates how we 'sense and move'. The somatic system is constantly active, as it coordinates movement instigated by the brain and transports sensory input to the brain. As such, it is at the core of the exploration function (see Figure 3.1).

A second system, the **sympathetic nervous system**, connects with our organs and glands and activates them to bring about a coordinated response to a perceived need for vigorous action. Its activation can work very quickly as an emergency response or build up over time to make us faster, stronger and more effective ('Go' or 'Fight or Flight'!). As you can see in Figure 3.1, this is a core function of our system. If you've ever crossed the street and suddenly had to run to save your life, you will know what the sympathetic response feels like. You may have stood on the pavement on the other side with your heart racing, panting, perhaps perspiring, and your knees trembling. On seeing the danger, the sympathetic nervous system would have accelerated your heart and breathing, increasing your blood pressure, and sent messages to the adrenal gland to produce adrenaline for the bloodstream to pump to the muscles to make you stronger and faster.

While sympathetic activity includes other aspects such as dilation of the pupils and suppression of digestion, the energising aspect is the essence. Being in the grip of the sympathetic response can be both empowering and overpowering and even stressful (Selye, 1956). Some theorists have connected sympathetic activation with the 'vitality' we might display (Stern, 2010). Others have emphasised that our efforts to perform tasks under pressure at an optimal level depend very much on how we learn to control our sympathetic response. Too much activation or 'arousal' – a synonymous term often used – might interfere with complex activities (Yerkes and Dodson, 1908). We would intuitively mistrust an overly activated, aroused or excited surgeon because we would suspect that this excitement might interfere with the controlled performance of an operation. You must remember that the sympathetic response is 'autonomic', and cannot be turned on and off at will, although we may learn to gain a certain degree of control. For example, to prepare for emergency interventions such as cardiopulmonary resuscitation (CPR) you can practise wilfully slowing down hurried movements, controlling your own breathing, and finding ways of stopping racing thoughts.

Scenario: Stop running around

In a chaotic Emergency Department (ED) of a major hospital ambulances are lining up outside unable to offload their patients. Inside there are waiting times for all except the most acute emergencies. All staff are running around to complete their tasks and making sure they keep an eye on the most urgent matters. At one point the nurse in charge makes a point of telling all staff to stop running. She explains that as we try to be faster our activation levels put us at risk of making more mistakes. Also, if one person runs, that triggers the same sense of urgency in others and in the end we may all be out of control. Do you agree?

The **parasympathetic nervous system** does the opposite of what the sympathetic nervous system does. Through a network of neural connections it facilitates relaxing, taking it easy and having our dinner ('Slow Down' or 'Rest and Digest'!). This is a core function of the human system and that of most animals (see Figure 3.1). Feeling very tired, sleepy, lazy or satiated after a meal are signals that your parasympathetic system is taking over. It includes slowing down of heart rate and breathing, reduction of muscle tone, and activation of the digestive system. It allows us to rest and recover and replenish our mental and physical resources. In the same way that the sympathetic nervous system protects us through the fight or flight response, the parasympathetic system safeguards against overburdening our system and coordinates 'refuelling'. Patients in hospitals often spend a lot of time in bed and therefore parasympathetic activity may be dominant. However, if they are anxious or nervous it is also possible that they are experiencing a lot of sympathetic activity. Lying in bed in such a state is unpleasant.

It is important to realise that, while the two systems are antagonistic, they can both be at work at a low level to control our activation levels in a range of activities. Typically the parasympathetic system takes over when the need for vigorous activity has passed, in order to slow us down. Sometimes it does this quite suddenly. For some of us, seeing blood leads to an instinctive fear reaction and a sympathetic response, which is immediately followed by a parasympathetic reaction that can be strong enough to significantly reduce the blood flow to the brain. This makes us faint.

Please do Activity 3.2 to check that you understand the peripheral nervous system and can apply your knowledge.

Activity 3.2 *Critical thinking*

Which part(s) of the peripheral nervous system would you expect to be most essential in the following activities? Discuss in detail (correct answers may include more than one part).

	Somatic	Sympathetic	Parasympathetic
1. Panicking.			
2. Trying to eat a meal during stressful work.			
3. Feeling pain.			
4. Being very angry.			
5. Burning your mouth and dropping your cup.			
6. Being on a quiet nightshift.			
7. Feeling stressed.			
8. Feeling 'sooo relaxed'.			
9. Giving birth.			
10. Performing CPR.			

An outline answer is provided at the end of the chapter.

Central nervous system

Our **central nervous system** consists of spine and brain. They are connected at the bottom of the skull at the back of our necks at a point often referred to as the brainstem.

The **spinal cord** includes a dual pathway of neural connections to and from the brain and is protected by the vertebral column. The three peripheral nervous systems all branch out from the spine. The spine is therefore the main connection between the peripheral nervous systems and the brain. While the spine is largely subservient to the brain, transmitting messages back and forth, it does also provide certain reflex responses before commands from the brain are given. A good example is the withdrawal of hands or feet from hot or sharp surfaces. If you step on to a nail, the spine receives the neural signal and immediately sends the message back to the muscles in foot and leg to lift the foot. If you touch a hot plate with your fingers, the spine will instantly give the command to withdraw the hand. This takes place before the information reaches the brain. Thus, important time is saved which helps limit tissue damage. Lack of voluntary control over these reflexes needs to be taken into account when potentially painful interventions or treatment are started with patients.

The **brain** is a complex information-processing unit the size of a grapefruit encased by the skull. Without the skull it looks a bit like a head of cauliflower, with a small cauliflower looking out from underneath on the rear side. It contains various types of neurons with different functions and different sizes. Estimates of the number of neurons in the brain vary from 86–110 billion, with many more support cells (glia) involved in various and not yet fully understood functions. Most of these neurons have many connections with other neurons. This mindboggling complexity allows for patterns of activation that facilitate the intricate coordination and command centre necessary to control and run the human system. The way many neurons are positioned in the brain is such that the cell bodies (soma) are often on the outside of the brain (cerebral cortex). This shows as grey matter. In contrast the myelin covered axons that branch off from the cell bodies to the inside of the brain look whitish (white matter).

To build up your understanding of the brain we have presented its structure in three overarching units (see Figure 3.2). This division was originally proposed by Paul MacLean as a way of presenting the evolutionary history of the brain. The 'triune brain' (MacLean and Kral, 1973) distinguishes between hindbrain (reptilian brain), limbic system or sub-cortical brain (mammal brain) and cerebrum (human or thinking brain). It is a sensible division because the three units show essential functional differences.

The **hindbrain**, on top of the spine at the back of the neck, contains structures that are essential to core bodily functions, such as coordination, balance, heartbeat, breathing, sleep patterns and other autonomous functions. In terms of the evolution of the brain this part is the oldest and, in its present organisation, very similar to the corresponding part of the brain in reptiles; hence its nickname the 'reptilian brain'. Severe damage to the hindbrain leads to instant death because breathing and heartbeat will cease. On top of the hindbrain we find the midbrain, which provides a waystation between hindbrain and the central section of the brain, the sub-cortical forebrain.

The **sub-cortical forebrain** contains the limbic system. This section of the brain consists of several modules with core coordinating functions that we have in common with other mammals (basic emotions, motivation, sexual excitement, care for offspring, memory encoding and decoding, hunger, etc.). What is often called the mammal or emotional brain is essential to ensure that we survive, reproduce and take care of our offspring. Pleasure centres are also situated partly in the sub-cortical area. This part of the brain does not produce complex thinking but immediate needs, motivations and urges. Unmodulated activity in the limbic system is perhaps best represented by how dogs behave. Think of how you come home to an overenthusiastic dog who slobbers up food and water without reservation and, when you have subsequently taken him for a walk, can't restrain himself when seeing another dog, while protectively barking and growling at anyone considered to pose a threat.

Around and on top of the sub-cortical forebrain we find the **cerebrum (or cerebral cortex)**. This part of our brain produces the typically human features such as complex thinking and understanding, problem solving, language, mathematical understanding, visual and auditory processing, complex motor skills, etc. The cerebrum produces our conscious thinking processes and is therefore nicknamed the thinking brain. Most intentional activities have their origin in the cerebrum. The cerebrum is the part of our brain that is most uniquely human. Its size, relative to the rest of the brain, is bigger in humans than in any other animal. The cerebrum helps us strategise and make plans, and is essential to regulate (and often suppress) emotions and urges generated in the subcortical forebrain. In contrast with a dog, our cerebrum is bigger and highly effective at moderating expressions of attraction and affection. We have table manners instead of gobbling up our food, and stop ourselves from always doing what comes to mind first. Most overarching functions in Figure 3.1 are at least partly processed in the cerebrum.

Concept summary: Pleasure and pain in the brain

Pleasure centres. In research with rats in the 1950s it was discovered that they were prepared to repeat pressing a lever continuously if this was paired with electrical stimulation of the brain (Olds, 1956) in the limbic system (sub-cortical forebrain). They liked it so much that if given the choice between this stimulation and food, they choose the stimulation. As a result they neglected eating, which led to starvation. The human pleasure experience is more complex and involves several pathways in both limbic system and cerebrum. Nonetheless, we can also be slaves to pleasure. Both when we are in love or under the influence of addictive drugs, the pleasure centres are flooded with dopamine, which intensifies the pleasure experience and reduces motivation to do anything else.

Pain centres. How we process pain is highly complex and involves several areas in the spine, hindbrain, sub-cortical forebrain and cerebrum. Interestingly, there are commonalities in the way in which pain and pleasure are processed and the locations in which this takes place. This goes some way to explaining how pain and pleasure may cancel each other out (Leknes and Tracey, 2008) and sometimes coincide. Itch and pain are also largely antagonistic in the brain, which explains why scratching reduces itch (Ikoma *et al.*, 2006). Moreover, this provides pleasure too! Furthermore, there is overlap between brain processes involved in 'physical' and 'mental' pain (Eisenberger and Lieberman, 2004). Finally, the (top of the) spine contains a pain modulating unit that functions as a gate that can open and close under the influence of emotions, distraction, relaxation, and rubbing around the area where the pain originates. We'll come back to this in more detail in Chapter 9 (see Gate Theory of Pain (Katz and Rosenbloom, 2015; Melzack and Wall, 1967)).

The integrated brain

Our brain operates to a large extent in an integrated way, which is facilitated by connections between most modules within the brain. For most activities of high complexity several parts of the brain are involved. Here are a few examples.

> *Movement:* for movement we need the motor cortex and somatosensory cortex (cerebrum), conveniently located alongside each other, but also the coordination networks in the cerebellum (hindbrain).
>
> *Talking:* to have a conversation we need our language centres, in the left hemisphere of the cerebrum. We also use the motor cortex (cerebrum) and cerebellum (hindbrain) to coordinate the movement of mouth, lips and tongue to produce speech. In addition, we need our auditory cortex (cerebrum) to understand what the other person is saying and to hear our own speech, and we need our hippocampus (sub-cortical forebrain) to help remember what is said and the amygdala (sub-cortical forebrain) to respond to the emotional aspect of the conversation.

In addition to collaborative neural activity, different parts of the brain may sometimes propagate contradictory responses or interfere with each other.

> *Being in love:* when you are 'in love' you may be motivated to a large extent by sub-cortical emotions. When you find out that the person you are in love with has political opinions that are opposite to yours, your cerebrum may tell you not to pursue it further. Funnily enough, this may not alter your feelings as dictated by sub-cortical sexual attraction. There may be an internal battle, and it is by no means a foregone conclusion which part of your brain will win.
>
> *Automated* versus *wilful movement:* when you run up the stairs you rely on your hindbrain (cerebellum) for coordination. This takes place automatically. If you start thinking about how you do it, your cerebrum tries to take over the coordination. How long until you will fall?
>
> *Overexcitement:* sometimes planned activities are sabotaged by overexcitement. Let's say you are nervous because you need to demonstrate your injection skills as part of an exam. Your cerebrum will produce the knowledge of how to do it and your sub-cortical forebrain may ensure that you are motivated but, perhaps, it is overdoing it and produces feelings of anxiety that, in turn, may lead to over-stimulation of the sympathetic nervous system, which may have a negative impact on fine motor skills and impede your handling of the injection needle (hindbrain).

The following exercise will allow you to explore examples of how different parts of the brain initiate and/or interact in common examples (Activity 3.3). It will provide you with a superior insight into how the brain operates.

Activity 3.3 — ***Critical thinking***

In which part(s) of the brain would you expect the most essential processing to take place in order to enable the following activities? Discuss dominant activity and debate in detail (the correct answer is often more than one part). At this point you may want to review your knowledge of the brain, using a physiology text or the Internet.

continued . . .

continued . . .

	Hindbrain	Sub-cortical Forebrain	Cerebrum
1. Greeting a new patient			
2. Feeling hungry, but you have to wait to eat			
3. Performing CPR			
4. Updating a patient's chart			
5. Changing a patient's position in bed			
6. Understanding a patient's emotions			
7. Feeling afraid			
8. Watching television			
9. Finding babies 'soooooo cute'			
10. Feeling 'wide awake but exhausted' after a nightshift			

An outline answer is provided at the end of the chapter.

Left and right brain

It is important to realise that from the hindbrain upwards almost all sections of the brain have a left and right part which, while similar in general function, can be different in specific aspects. Elaborate connections allow for integral rather than separate operation of these left and right parts. For the cerebrum, the left and right hemispheres are connected by a neural super highway called the **corpus callosum**. Funnily enough, we have our wires crossed in the sense that where the hemispheres correspond with our senses or body parts, it is always the opposite-side hemisphere that connects to a particular side of the body or sense. So, left ear and eye corresponds with the right hemisphere in the brain, while the right arm or leg is processed in the left hemisphere, etc. The other most important distinction is that in the majority of people the left hemisphere of the cerebrum processes language, while the right hemisphere is more involved in visual spatial orientation. This goes a long way to explaining why people who prefer to use a map have very little appreciation of people who prefer verbal instructions: they use different parts of their brain.

Plasticity and development of the brain

Our brains develop throughout our lives and their connections are in constant flux. This is called 'plasticity'. This facilitates one of our main overarching functions – 'adaptation' (see Figure 3.1), which enables us to become and maintain expertly adapted to the lives we lead. In childhood, expansion dominates (see Chapter 4) and then, later, reduction through pruning in neural connections occurs. These processes together help us learn and process information in diverse and effective ways. There is also evidence that there is a gradual development throughout our lives towards more dominant activity in the front and upper parts of the brain (Davis *et al.*, 2008). This facilitates more control through our thinking (and perhaps wisdom) when we get older. In late adulthood, development tends to stall and, not uncommonly these days, the ravages of dementia make life difficult. We'll address this in more detail in Chapter 4.

Case study: The impact of a shocking experience

Maria is attending her first day on the medical ward in a general hospital as a nursing student. Just after the patients have received their morning tea, Maria enters one of the six-bedded areas. She strolls past the first bed and, as she reaches the second patient, she sees what looks like a grey corpse. Instinctively she freezes on the spot. She can't speak, is paralysed by fear and becomes aware of trembling and rapid breathing. Fortunately her mentor was right behind her and raises the alarm. Attempts to revive the patient are unsuccessful and, when working alongside her mentor later that morning, Maria finds that she is still shaking. Later on she calms down but she is still upset, trying to make sense of it all, and wonders what would have happened if they had arrived earlier at the patient's bed. At the end of the day she is really tired.

Can you map out the activity in Maria's brain and nervous system during and after the events? What support should Maria receive?

An outline response is provided at the end of the chapter.

The chemistry of psychology

It is uncertain whether we have done the right thing by presenting the psychology of the nervous system without focusing more on the chemical aspect. This may have created the impression that thinking, emotions and behaviour are essentially coordinated only by electrical sources. This is far from the truth. The core of the neural response, the action potential, involves a flow of chemicals in and out of the axon, mainly sodium and potassium, and communication from one neuron to another is done by other chemicals – 'transmitters'. While the body produces these transmitters, their production can be influenced by nutrition, activity levels and drugs. There is also a whole system of hormonal communication within us, the endocrine system, which interacts with the nervous system but also has its own complex functions. It would leave a significant hole in your understanding of how communication takes place within our system if we did not address this.

Like the nervous system, the **endocrine system** is a signalling system and, while the way in which it works is very different, it is equally essential to how we live our lives. Without endocrine stimulation we would not grow and develop, and we would not be hungry, digest our food nor have sexual appetite, we would not sleep, nor be fully awake and active, etc. It is safe to say that there are very few activities that do not have a hormonal involvement. The nervous system sends information very quickly, and responses are mostly short-lived. In contrast, endocrine responses may last from minutes, to hours or even days or weeks. While the nervous system works through a combination of electrical (dry) and transmission activity (wet), the endocrine system relies on the messenger function of molecules that are first and foremost produced by endocrine glands (pituitary, pineal, adrenal, thymus, thyroid, pancreas, ovaries, testes) and that are secreted into blood vessels to travel to where they are used to promote specific activities. Of particular importance is the master gland, the pituitary, which conveniently hangs from the bottom of the hypothalamus (in the sub-cortical forebrain), which controls general activity level, hunger, digestion and sexual activity. This forms the main point of contact between the nervous system and the endocrine system. The great advantage of this is that essential neural and endocrine activity can be coordinated more effectively. For instance, the fight or flight response, which originates in the hypothalamus, creates a synchronous response in the pituitary, which in turn leads to joint stimulation of the adrenal gland and the sympathetic nervous system. This is often referred to as the 'hypothalamus–pituitary–adrenal gland axis', which is essential to how we experience stress (see Chapter 8).

The complexity of the endocrine system is comparable to the nervous system and, like the nervous system, the endocrine glands affect each other and generate joint responses. The endocrine system often seems to work as a 'fertiliser' that enlarges mood swings (Diehl and Gershon, 1992), increases pleasure and pain, and promotes or suppresses sexual interest and activity. Overall, endocrine functions seem to make a meaningful candidate for further psychological research. The domino effects of unbalanced hormone levels would suggest that this type of research will be of a high complexity. At present it is still in its infancy, but it is gaining attention.

Research summary: The secret workings of hormones

During ovulation women undergo hormonal changes due to **oestrogen** release that affect how they prepare for a night out (Baker and Bellis, 1995). Baker and Bellis demonstrated this in an interesting study in which they asked women who entered a night club to provide a urine sample to establish whether or not they were ovulating and then they took a picture of them after they had taken off their coats. They found that the extent of 'flesh' shown was higher in women who were ovulating. The women were not aware that their choice of dress had been affected by their hormones, but Baker and Bellis theorised that this may well be rooted in an adaptation that combines the chance to get pregnant with looking available. Related studies on nightclub behaviour showed similar effects on wearing make-up and preparedness to dance (Guéguen, 2009; Grammer *et al.*, 2004).

The impact of **testosterone** on the brain in both men and women is a rich source of debate. There is evidence to suggest that being in leadership positions leads to higher concentrations of testosterone in the brain, which in turn leads to more authoritarian behaviour. This makes us unreasonably bossy. Many world leaders and managers have been affected by this, which often made them lose perspective on the issues they were facing (Robertson, 2012).

Chapter 3

Sensation and perception

Having introduced how we process information in the nervous system and the endocrine system, it is now time to look at how we gather information about our world (sensation) and how the brain makes sense of it (perception). **Sensation** takes place in eyes, ears, tongue, nose and skin and muscle tissue (Figure 3.3). All the information gathered by the senses makes its way to the brain. The processing in the brain is called **perception** and is focused on giving meaning and organising our multiple sensations. It takes place in separate specialised areas of the cortex after having been routed through the thalamus to allow cross referencing between the different types of sensory information. Smell is an exception and enters the brain via the olfactory bulb before being routed directly to the olfactory cortex.

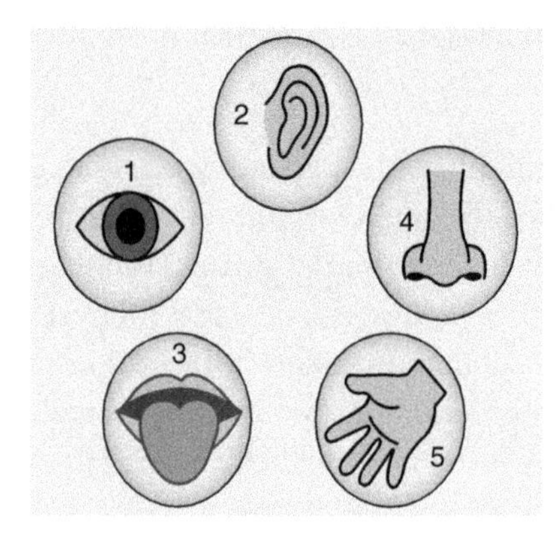

1) Visual system (SIGHT)
2) Auditory system (HEARING)
3) Gustatory system (TASTE)
4) Olfactory system (SMELL)
5) Cutaneous senses and the vestibular system (TOUCH, TEMPERATURE, PAIN, BODY and HEAD POSITION AND MOVEMENT)

Figure 3.3: The five senses

Sensation

The senses provide us with detailed information about our environment and our own body. Each of our senses is highly sensitive to detail and processes a wide range of the type of stimulus it records. Nonetheless, each of the senses has a threshold below which the neurons do not fire. These thresholds are affected by the intensity of stimuli we receive. When we've listened to very loud music, our ears are subsequently less responsive. If we've looked at something in very bright daylight we have difficulty seeing things in the shade. The senses adapt to a certain extent to the frequency and intensity of the stimuli. We tend to emphasise the importance of what we see and hear and there is still a lot we don't know in regard to how smell or taste affects us.

Overall, the effectiveness of the senses differs between people. Sharp vision and hearing provides us with pleasure and a sense of control. Unfortunately, our senses are subject to wear and tear during our lifetime. To a certain extent the brain can compensate for minor reductions in sensory effectiveness, but it can become debilitating. Hearing loss hinders essential information gathering and inhibits social contact, which can be an isolating factor (Weinstein and Ventry, 1982). Particularly in old age this can accelerate the ageing process and contribute to dementia (Lin *et al.*, 2011). The same can be said for diminished vision. Again, in old age being unable to orientate oneself effectively, watch television, or read a book leads to people losing these faculties and subsequently their appetite for life. Of course, glasses and hearing aids can make up for much of these losses, but they do have limitations. Having said this, recent technological and medical advances are giving new hope to those severely affected.

Case study: Dealing with sensory limitations

Martin (age 65) was recently diagnosed with melanoma of his right eye and has just undergone radioactive plaque therapy, under general anaesthetic, to treat his eye cancer. The result of this is that he must wear an eye patch for a few days and his vision in that eye will be affected in the short term at least (double vision, blurredness and loss of vision). While this takes place, it transpires that the batteries in his hearing aid have run down and there are no immediate replacements. Without this he hears very little. Although it is important to foster his independence and recovery, think about the possible problems he may encounter and what you can do to help. Write your answers down.

An outline response is provided at the end of the chapter.

Perception

The function of the senses is to receive and transform information from the outside and inside world into neural signals that can be processed by the brain. In a way it is only after our brain has made sense of these neural signals – we call this **perception** – that we actually see, hear, taste, smell and feel. More than anything, perception is a process of selection, highlighting and picking up regularities and irregularities in the chaotic sensory signals we receive. Psychological research on perception has focused to a large extent on vision, but similar principles can be applied to understand how we make sense of sound, taste and smell. Perception is partly learned and develops as a result of experience with stimulation from the senses. This means that, for instance, if a child is born blind and its eyesight can be restored at age ten there is the added complication that the brain has not developed to process vision and therefore the child will still not be able to see.

Fundamental perceptual principles

Our brain is equipped with the ability to establish constancies in the visual signals we receive. Our heads and eyes are moving and thereby sending information about our environment in a rather chaotic fashion to the visual cortex. However, the different neural layers have an uncanny ability to establish which aspects have remained the same. At its most basic level our brains correct for size, shape and brightness.

Size constancy allows us to recognise that an object when seen from close by, is the same as when observed from a distance. We take it for granted that we recognise a bed regardless of whether we stand close to it or far away; however, we need to realise that our brain needs to make the comparison and confirm the constancy in order to confidently experience our environment.

Shape constancy helps us recognise the same object even if it is seen from a different angle. Thus we will recognise a table or a bed regardless of the angle from which we see it. Our ability to mentally rotate objects helps with this process.

Brightness constancy relates to the fact that objects are recognised as the same regardless of the amount of light that falls on them. We essentially correct for the saturation of light and colour in our visual field. Of course, some of this correction takes place through the contraction and opening of our iris, but our brains provide the recognition of constancies regardless of brightness differences.

Essentially 'size, shape and brightness constancy rescue us from a confusing world in which objects would seem to shrink and grow, change shape as if made of rubber, and light up and fade like neon lamps' (Coon, 2004, p. 215).

Early in the twentieth century the **Gestalt psychology** movement provided us with a number of insights that are still valid. They were specifically interested in how our perceptual system turned the separate neural input into the perception of 'wholes' (or Gestalts). A series of laws were formulated (Wertheimer, 1923) that reflected visual processing (see Figure 3.4). In this way we are able to organise stimuli in meaningful ways, distinguish an object of interest from its background, and complete partial visual information. The Gestalt principles also include preferences and expectations of symmetry and 'good form'.

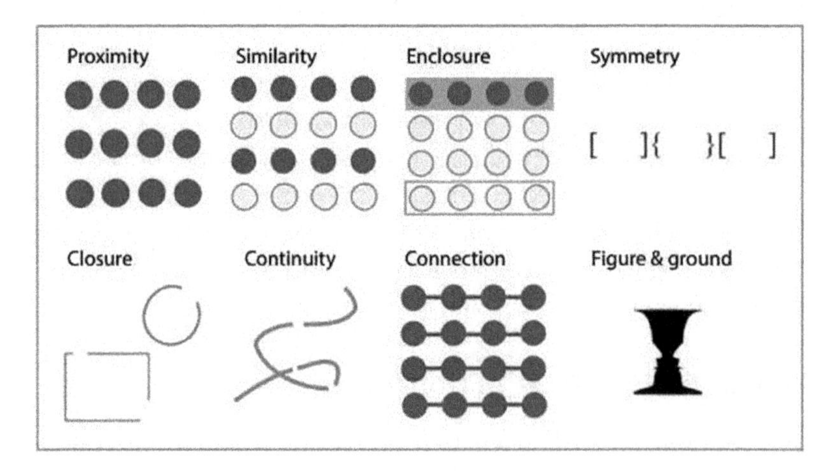

Figure 3.4: Gestalt principles of perception

We must realise that our sight and that of other mammals has developed and adapted to make sense of the world in ways that aid our survival. For instance, figure and ground perception is particularly astute when an object is moving. Depth perception is also a particular strength. Having two eyes helps, but visual cues for distance such as the expected size of objects, their overlap, the clarity of objects, light and shadow, allow us to be highly accomplished at estimating the distance between ourselves and objects of interest. A patient who has one eye covered will have to activate such monocular cues for distance, because binocular cues are not available. Initially they are at risk of estimating distance wrongly. Interestingly, proper depth perception seems to develop in infants when they start crawling (Gibson and Walk, 1960).

It is essential to appreciate that we were adapted to process information in a three-dimensional world. Whenever we see something in a two-dimensional depiction, our brains automatically look for cues to read it as a three dimensional stimulus. This is a process that includes considerable risk of making mistakes. Look for 'perceptual illusions' on the Internet. For auditory perception similar principles apply. Sounds are also subject to Gestalt principles similar to size, shape and brightness constancies, in the guise of loudness, pitch and timbre (Todorovic, 2008). As a result we recognise the voices of people we know, regardless of how loudly they speak, what they say, and whether their voices are near, far, or muffled, as on the phone.

Combining different sensory modes is facilitated by the brain. Because all but our smell is routed through the thalamus, this allows the combination and cross referencing of multi-modal sensory information at the earliest point of entry in the brain. In some people this leads to the experience of synaesthesia. They can 'see' sounds in colours, or 'hear' the voice of a person they see, etc. This facility is useful because we can call up visual imagery when we only hear the sound of something that concerns us and the other way around.

Higher order perception

While we have an instinctive orienting response (processed by reticular formation in hindbrain and midbrain) that automatically orients us towards loud sounds and the direction of sudden movement, much of our attention is based on what we are especially interested in at a particular moment. Once we pay attention, more elaborate and refined perceptual processes are activated. Higher order perception makes use of expectations based on earlier experience stored in memory and conceptual understanding of our world and ourselves.

We are affected considerably by the context in which we see, hear or feel something. In a hospital you expect to see doctors and nurses and if someone puts on a white coat and hangs a stethoscope around the neck, we are easily deceived. Equally we tend to look for signs of illness in our patient, because that is what we expect in our line of work. This emphasis has an important impact on what we highlight and what we ignore. Seeing a red blotch somewhere in a hospital will alert a nurse because the suspicion that it is blood will be activated. In contrast, a bright green or blue spot may go more or less unnoticed because it may not generate instant concerns. Psychologists have noted that when we examine a situation with a particular expectation, we often jump to conclusions, because we naturally try to confirm the correctness of our expectation. This is called **confirmation bias**. We are most at risk of making this mistake when we draw conclusions from a general principle, referred to as 'top-down processing'. The alternative is bottom-up processing, which tends to occur when we try to make sense of our world on the basis of many observations and reach conclusions only after detailed efforts to examine the stimuli. A diagnostic interview is generally set up to allow the diagnosis to emerge from the information and is made only after enough indications are pointing in a particular direction.

Activity 3.4 — *Critical thinking*

Read the scenario which follows. It contains six elements that could lead to false preceptions. Can you identify them all? If you were the nurse, what would you do?

It is a normal day in the children's hospital. Doctor Hansen has done her rounds and tells you that she suspects that one child who has just arrived is suffering from Attention Deficit and Hyperactivity Disorder (ADHD). Later that day you realise that one of the light bulbs in the room where you sort the medication has popped. One of the heart monitors is malfunctioning and keeps beeping although the patient is fine. You are reading a diagram that explains the use of a new piece of equipment but it seems cluttered and you can't make much sense of it. When your colleagues come back from their lunch they are very relaxed and chatty. Some of the children are very loud and you have difficulty hearing what else is going on. When you enter a six-bed ward you see five children in good form. Of the sixth child you can only see an arm. The rest seems to be covered by blankets and pillows.

An outline answer is provided at the end of the chapter.

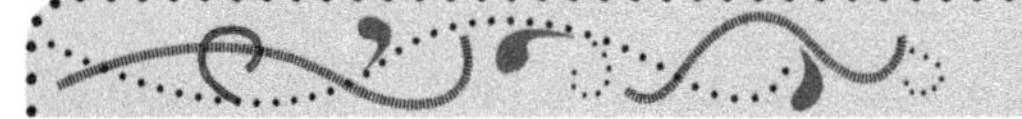

Chapter summary

- Our core psychological functions have evolved to facilitate survival and reproduction and the activities that contribute to this.
- This is reflected in the functions of the nervous system as highlighted in Figure 3.1:
  - fight or flight – sympathetic nervous system;
  - rest and digest – parasympathetic nervous system;
  - sense and move – somatic nervous system;
  - balance, coordination, autonomous functions – hind brain;
  - curiosity, hunger, fear, aggression, attraction, love, attachment, care – motivated initially in sub-cortical forebrain;
  - overarching functions – cerebrum and combination of brain sections.
- The endocrine system has an often hidden impact on our behaviour. Examples of its influence on psychology are ubiquitous.
- Sensation and perception are essential functions. We must beware that we are subject to sensory and perceptual illusions.
- It is important for nurses to be aware of the complexity of the functions and mechanisms addressed here in order to understand themselves, patients and colleagues, and how care is facilitated and hindered.
- After reading this chapter you will hopefully have a better idea of why we function in the way we do, why we are aware of some activities while other activities seem to take place automatically, and why we often find it difficult to control our emotions or strong urges.

Activities: brief outline answers

Activity 3.2 (see page 41)

The somatic system is involved in all examples. It is a matter of identifying sympathetic or parasympathetic dominance: 1) panicking – sympathetic; 2) trying to eat a meal during stressful work – parasympathetic and sympathetic compete; 3) feeling pain – somatic, sympathetic if it upsets you; 4) being very angry – sympathetic; 5) burning your mouth and dropping your cup – somatic, sympathetic if is upsets you; 6) being on a quiet nightshift – risk of too much parasympathetic activity; 7) feeling stressed – sympathetic; 8) feeling 'sooo relaxed' – parasympathetic; 9) giving birth – complex interaction between all three systems; 10) performing CPR – sympathetic.

Activity 3.3 (see page 44)

Hindbrain is always active in the background. It is important to see the difference between cerebral and sub-cortical (limbic) dominance. 1) Greeting a new patient – cerebral, but you will also have a sub-conscious sub-cortical response; 2) Feeling hungry, but you have to wait to eat – sub-cortical, with cerebral effort to distract yourself; 3) Performing CPR – collaboration between all three sections; 4) Updating a patient's chart – cerebral; 5) Changing a patient's position in bed – cerebral and hindbrain – your cerebrum gives instructions, your hindbrain helps coordinate your movements; the more automated your efforts the more the hindbrain dominates; 6) Understanding a patient's emotions – subcortical, cerebrum; 7) Feeling afraid – sub-cortical – cerebrum can help reduce or intensify fear; 8) Watching television – cerebrum, sub-cortical – when you are affected by what you watch there is sub-cortical activity; 9) Finding babies 'soooooo cute' – sub-cortical; 10) Feeling 'wide awake but exhausted' after a night shift – hindbrain – you experience contradictory signals to sleep and to be awake.

Case study: The impact of a shocking experience (see page 46)

Her subcortical (limbic) response in the brain will have been very intense, leading to a strong sympathetic nervous system reaction. Her cerebrum will have been really busy afterwards trying to come to terms with what happened and her own reaction. The energy needed for this is draining and will trigger a parasympathetic reaction. It is not uncommon for experiences involving death to have an intense impact which can, in some cases, lead to post traumatic stress (PTSD) later on. Some form of debriefing may help Maria process what has happened.

Case study: Dealing with sensory limitations (see page 49)

He will have difficulty moving around without bumping into objects. He will feel isolated because he is not hearing much. He may feel disoriented and upset. He may try to hide his helplessness but needs assistance moving around (at first). The nurse may need to be alert during these temporary sensory limitations and ensure that all communication is understood.

Activity 3.4 (see page 52)

Doctor Hansen is perhaps a bit quick on the ADHD diagnosis and may be subject to confirmation bias. (1) Bad lighting (2) is an important risk factor in medication mistakes. Continued alarm signals (3) need to be addressed at all costs, because true alarms will not be responded to if this is a frequent problem. Unclear instructions (4) in manuals of equipment are a common source of accidents. A high baseline of noise (5) drowns out potential distress signals. Seeing an arm may lead to the assumption that there is a whole child (principle of closure) (6). It may be important to check.

Further reading

Ward, J. (2015) *The student's guide to cognitive neuroscience* (3rd Ed.). Hove: Psychology Press.

There are many good introductions to cognitive neuroscience but this one is particularly accessible.

Melmed, S., Polonsky, K. S., Larsen, P. R. and Kronenberg, H. M. (2015) *Williams textbook of endocrinology* (13th Ed.). Philadelphia, PA: Elsevier Health Sciences.

This text is considered the gold standard of endocrinology.

DeLucia, P. R. and Levulis, S. J. (2015) 'Basics of sensation and perception with an eye toward application' in Boehm-Davis, Deborah A. (Ed.), Durso, Francis T., Lee, John D. (Ed.) (2015). *APA handbook of human systems integration. APA handbooks in psychology* (pp. 229–245). Washington, DC: American Psychological Association.

The emphasis on application makes this a particularly useful text on sensation and perception.

Useful websites

https://www.youtube.com/watch?v=q_5myLhhzwE

This link connects to the BBC programme 'The Human Brain'. There are many other videos online that explain how the brain works in highly effective ways. Watching these is an effective use of your time.

https://en.wikipedia.org/wiki/Perception

Wikipedia's entry on perception provides significant background.

https://www.youtube.com/watch?v=9-OQbo_aWbA

Here is a YouTube video illustrating perceptual illusions. YouTube has many relevant videos. Use keywords such as: perceptual illusion, visual illusion, sensory illusion, Ames Room, auditory or audio illusion.

https://www.youtube.com/watch?v=kzo45hWXRWU

This presentation demonstrates auditory illusions. Look for Diana Deutsch for more.

Chapter 4
How we develop and how we learn

Chapter aims

After reading this chapter you will be able to:

- explain how the human system develops and how genetic and environmental factors interact to bring about this process;
- understand lifespan development and its implications for providing care to people in different age groups;
- understand the four mechanisms of learning: association (in particular classical conditioning), consequences (operant learning), observation/imitation (modelling) and understanding (cognitive learning);
- apply the four mechanisms of learning in nursing and health care.

Caring for a baby is very different from caring for an adolescent or a younger or older adult. Nurses adapt their care and support according to the age and developmental phase of the patient. To do so in appropriate ways it is essential to understand how humans develop and change during their life course. This includes the interaction between our genetic predispositions and what is learned in life. Furthermore, it is essential that you understand the mechanisms whereby we learn. We discriminate between learning through association (in particular classical conditioning), consequences (operant learning), observation/imitation (modelling) and understanding (cognitive learning). Practical examples will guide you in developing your understanding of how nursing skills are acquired and how you can use and pass on your knowledge of health- and illness-related principles, skills and behaviours to people in your care.

Development: nature–nurture interactions

We develop from conception to death according to a genetic blueprint that unfolds step by step in a pattern that is similar for all humans, but shows considerable variation between individuals. This development will take place in response to stimulation from the environment and our own activities, which trigger the genes to be active or be dormant. From within the cells genes orchestrate growth, progress, and eventually ageing using intricate biological messenger systems. Overall, development is the combined result of our inherited nature represented by our DNA and the impact of how we are raised, educated and our experiences in the world. It is important to realise that one cannot do without the other: nature and nurture interact and one cannot be expressed without the other. Before we get started in earnest with this chapter we would like to check something with you regarding your perspective on the nature<> nurture debate. We are sure you've heard of it. It is essentially about whether you believe we are mostly affected by the qualities we've inherited or by the way in which we were raised and educated.

Activity 4.1 *Reflection*

Please answer the following questions:

1. When someone is shy you assume he or she has always been shy.
   mostly true/mostly false
2. Children raised in foster families are still more like their birth parents.
   mostly true/mostly false
3. Prisoners are born with a lack of control over their impulses.
   mostly true/mostly false
4. People have a higher chance to get really old if their grandparents did.
   mostly true/mostly false
5. Mental illness is often hereditary.
   mostly true/mostly false
6. Smart people became smart because of a very good education.
   mostly true/mostly false
7. Drug addiction has its roots in upbringing and influences during adolescence.
   mostly true/mostly false
8. When you see people with amazing talents you assume they worked hard at them.
   mostly true/mostly false
9. When you see children misbehave you blame the parents' poor parenting.
   mostly true/mostly false
10. You can become anything you want in life as long as you put in an effort.
    mostly true/mostly false

Questions 1–5: Add a point for each 'mostly true' answer.
Questions 6–10: Add a point for each 'mostly false' answer.
Add up the scores. If you have 0-3 points you tend to consider 'nurture' more important; 4-6 points, you tend to appreciate both perspectives; 7-10 points, you consider human success and failure mostly as part of their 'nature'.

Development is a reciprocal and 'active' process

We are not passively waiting for the environment to affect us, we act. This is not only true for adults, but also for children. 'Children set their own development in motion' (p. 28) and 'children change their world even as it changes them' (Papalia *et al.*, 2004, p. 29). They seek out stimulation. They demand their parents' attention, initially by crying and cooing, and reward them with a smile when they feel nurtured or entertained. They are genetically prepared to cry when in discomfort. Likewise, parents are genetically programmed to find a baby's crying unbearable and to do anything to stop it. In fact, children manipulate their parents and other caregivers into caring for them and educating them, while parents are strongly inclined to attend and relate to their offspring. The evolutionary perspective on psychology emphasises that such interacting qualities ensure that children survive. Moreover, children's specific preferences and assets play an important role from early on in the kind of stimulation they receive and generate. For example, an outgoing child may beseech its parents for opportunities to be among other children, while a shy child may try to avoid such occasions (Kagan *et al.*, 1988). Within these situations other children and adults will communicate quite differently with the outgoing child as compared with the shy child, thereby turning the event into a very different experience. In general, it is difficult to predict the outcome of complex interactions between the child's traits, its behaviour, responses from others, the family, neighbourhood, school and wider cultural and social context. Much of this unfolds in how children play, individually and in interaction with others. Play is practice for life and crucial in child development.

Stage theories of development

Many theories of development emphasise a succession of stages or phases most people go through. These often coincide with the common denominators in life in the Western world, such as going to school at a particular age, having a family, working, and retirement. To a large extent our lives are 'scripted' and developmental theories tend to emphasise these scripted pathways. It is important to question the relevance of these theories when pathways in life do not follow a standard pattern or follow it at a different pace. For instance, being single or married sets people on very different life courses with very different roles to perform. Also, it probably says more about a person's development to know that they are married with children (and how old the children are) than to know whether they are in their 20s, 30s, or 40s. Similarly, we may discover more about a child by learning whether it has already been exposed to crèches and schooling than whether it is four or five years old. Another specific issue is that developmental stage theories of the past have become less applicable to contemporary ageing because we tend to live longer and remain fit longer. In short, while we will be presenting the most popular stage theories, it is important for you to maintain a critical perspective.

Spring in the brain

The tree in your garden undergoes a dramatic transformation in spring. Quite suddenly it starts to grow new branches, new shoots sprout, new leaves, new buds and, invisible to us, new roots. When a baby is born a similar transformation takes place in its brain. We call this 'Spring in the Brain', an idea inspired by Bruce Perry (Perry and Szalavitz, 2007). Suddenly, the 100 billion or so neurons in the brain start to develop more dendrites, terminal buttons and synapses. In your garden this development is stimulated by more sunlight and higher temperatures that, with some rain, will make nutrients in the soil accessible. In humans, nutrients are also needed, but it is stimulation through the senses that leads to this massive growth. This stimulation comes from the outside world and the activities in which the newborn engages.

This development is illustrated with the picture (Figure 4.1) of a small segment of an infant's brain as a neonate, at six months and after two years. This growth is essential to create a well-networked brain that will prepare the child to be effective in our complex world. A child that grows up in an

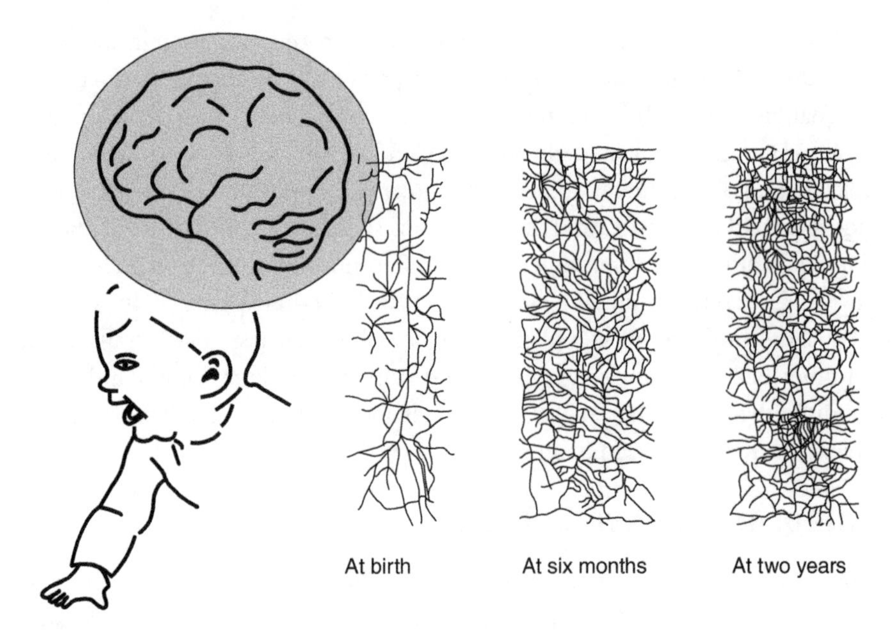

Figure 4.1: Spring in the brain (neural development in infants)

enriched environment, in which it receives lots of stimulation, attention, love, and opportunities to play and explore, is likely to develop a brain that will be fit for this world. However, if the child is neglected or deprived of important stimulation it will not develop the neural connectivity it needs. You need to realise that this is by no means common knowledge. Poor parenting skills are quite common and many parents are not aware that this may jeopardise their children's future (Perry, 2008). Evidence from follow-up research on children from orphanages, such as were common in Romania during the communist era, shows that lack of personal and physical contact with caregivers led to cognitive and behavioural deficits that could be traced to poor development in parts of the brain (Chugani *et al.*, 2001). Every now and again we hear about a child that has been kept in a basement or attic or perhaps lived in the wild ('feral children'), with catastrophic effects on their development. More often than not these children have developmental deficits that cannot be made up for later on in life (Perry and Szalavitz, 2007). You wonder how Romulus and Remus managed to found Rome (Bremmer, 1987) after having been raised by a wolf.

Case study: Developmental deprivation in hospital

Christopher is a two-year-old boy with cancer. He is well known to the staff on the children's ward where you are working due to several admissions over preceding months. Treatment is effective overall, but there have been setbacks that meant Christopher has spent weeks on end in the hospital. What are the developmental risks of prolonged hospital admissions for a two year old? What should nurses do to address these risks? What are your views on how often parents should visit? Should care at home be facilitated if possible? Write out your thoughts.

An outline response is provided at the end of the chapter.

Life span development

Prenatal development

Developmental theories used to start with birth. Today we know better. What happens in the first nine months in the womb is vital (Slade *et al.*, 2009). This does not mean that we fully understand all that affects development in the womb, but we know that the mother's behaviour and experiences affect the health and mental health of the foetus. Research has conclusively demonstrated that smoking, drinking alcohol, certain illnesses, stress and an overall unhealthy life style of the pregnant mother have a negative, sometimes lasting, impact on the child (Kaiser and Allen, 2008). In addition, we are wondering about the impact of stress. Psychologically pregnancy is a significant event for the mother-to-be and comes with anticipation, excitement, but also concerns. The birth of the child is often seen as a moment of crisis and stress for the mother (Kitzinger, 2006). Considering that the stress hormones in the mother's bloodstream also flow in the foetus' circulatory system, the stress of the mother is bound to impact the foetus/baby (Mulder *et al.*, 2002; Monk *et al.*, 2000; Lorenz, 1937). Research on this is still in its infancy, but the shared circulatory system and the fact that the foetus depends on the mother for its nutrients make it very clear that the health of mother and foetus have to be closely interlinked (Federenko and Wadhwa, 2004).

Childhood

After birth we distinguish the Neonatal period (first four weeks), which is a period of rapid development of just about all aspects. In terms of providing care, this is an intense period of monitoring all functions and responding to the baby's needs. Within psychology, 'infancy' is generally used to indicate the first two years in the child's life in which perhaps the most significant developments take place in motor skills, sensory perception, social interaction, communication and cognitive abilities. Any long-term nursing care would have to include providing stimulation to facilitate these developments.

The period from two to five years old is referred to as early childhood and more or less ends when the child goes to school. Middle childhood (from 6–11) more or less covers the primary school period in which the child grows towards independent functioning on most fronts.

One of the most important mechanisms to facilitate early development is **attachment**, or the affection and strong bond that develops between infant and caregiver (Weiten, 2010). Research by Lorenz on imprinting in birds such as ducks and geese (Lorenz, 1937) made us wonder whether such a process also takes place in humans. When a duckling comes out of the egg a rapid process takes place in the duckling's brain whereby the shape of what it sees first, that fits the description of a rounded life form, is imprinted in the brain. The duckling then proceeds to follow this shape wherever it goes. Normally this is the mother, of course. This is an adaptive response that guarantees protection and learning of all the things a duckling or gosling needs to know. Would human babies also imprint their mother in such an instant fashion? Evidence suggests it is a slower and less absolute process in humans. Erikson suggests that during the first year of life 'trust' develops (Erikson, 1959) as a reflection on the trustworthiness of the relationship with the caregivers. It is mostly at around six to eight months that infants start showing specific preference for main caregivers, usually the mother.

This attachment is normally precipitated by intense face-to-face contact (Volker *et al.*, 1999) and becomes stronger based on frequency of sensitive and responsive interactions including play (Leyendecker *et al.*, 1997). Empirical research to test attachment levels in the lab made use of the 'strange situation'. Mary Ainsworth let mothers and infants play in a room and observed the child's behaviour when the mother was called away for a brief period of time. Of particular interest was what happened on her return. 'Securely attached' infants were upset on her leaving but quickly calmed down once the mother returned. Those who were neither upset on her leaving nor seeking contact on their return were considered showing an 'avoidant attachment'. A third group showed distress on the mother leaving but were not easily consoled on her return. Their attachment was considered 'anxious-ambivalent' (Ainsworth *et al.*, 1978). Bowlby was among the first to suggest in the 1970s that a strong or secure attachment, particularly with both parents, was predictive of healthy adult development (Bowlby, 2005) including the ability to form intimate relationships later on in life. Attachment processes are strengthened by emerging fear of strangers and separation anxiety after the eighth month (Greenberg *et al.*, 1973). As a nurse it is important to be aware of these mechanisms and to find ways of overcoming fear of strangers and providing a substitute attachment during a child's stay in hospital.

Case study: Attachment

Hala is a new-born who is being nursed in the Neonatal ICU where you are working.

She has breathing difficulties following her birth and is diagnosed with transient tachypnoea of the new-born (TTN). This means she is breathing fast, she may have fluid on her lungs and she requires oxygen and respiratory support. She is being nursed in an incubator, being closely monitored and has a nasal mask supporting her breathing with positive airway pressure (Continuous Positive Airway Pressure (CPAP)). From our previous discussions on attachment, can you think of how nurses might promote mother, father and child bonding in this situation? Write your answers down.

An outline response is provided at the end of the chapter.

Parenting and schooling

Parenting and schooling have an important impact on development. Perspectives on what is good parenting have developed greatly over time. In tandem with schooling that is much more diverse and incorporates a much wider variety of knowledge and abilities, the average upbringing and education tends to facilitate high levels of academic and social proficiency in many of today's children. Perhaps most importantly the use of physical punishment as a means of disciplining children has gradually become less popular and is now outlawed in most Western countries, first in schools, but now also within the home. The reasoning behind this is manifold but generally includes that children need to feel safe to learn and develop well, that they learn better from rewards rather than punishment (see next section) and that it is undesirable to perpetuate physical and verbal aggression, because of the long-term negative impact on the child (Vissing *et al.*, 1991). A popular typology of **parenting styles** (Baumrind, 1971) distinguishes between 'authoritarian', 'permissive' and 'authoritative' parenting. The authoritarian style ('do as I say') is often considered to generate obedience, but there is evidence that children raised in this way in Britain turned out with lower social competence and conduct problems (Thompson *et al.*, 2003). In contrast, permissive parenting generates rebelliousness and chaos and lower levels of competence. The ideal perspective, authoritative parenting, in which the parents' authority is not imposed but, while rules are set, they are accepted and subject to negotiation and explanation, has been demonstrated to generate capable children in Western culture. Baumrind's typology has since been expanded with the 'uninvolved' parenting style (Maccoby, 1992), which is not desirable, and the principle of 'good enough parenting', which is heavily debated (Ramaekers and Suissa, 2012).

Considering the difficulty many parents have, it is understandable that there is support for the thought that they may not need to be perfect to generate a more or less effective upbringing. Meanwhile, the pressure of dealing with a variety of common disabilities such as attention deficit and hyperactivity disorder (ADHD) means that parents may be out of their depth and need assistance in the form of parenting skills training (Zwi *et al.*, 2011). Other common concerns today are the levels of on-screen (television, computer games) violence many children are exposed to, the lack of healthy nutrition, lack of physical exercise in many households, and the impact of bullying and exclusion in schools, which may compound behavioural problems in children.

Case study: Attention deficit and hyperactivity disorder (ADHD)

Joseph is an eight-year-old diagnosed with ADHD who is currently receiving support from the community mental health team. At a recent case conference the team became concerned about the parent-child relationship insofar as the mother seemed to be quite stressed about Joseph's behaviour and quite intolerant of some of his actions. Joseph is reluctant to speak about such issues, but the community mental health nurse, through her relationship with Joseph, gleans information that seems to indicate that his mother is using an authoritative parenting style and inflicting punishments such as locking him in his room. Consider the core of the issue and what action might be taken in this situation. Write your answers down.

An outline response is provided at the end of the chapter.

Cognitive and moral development

Jean Piaget (see Activity 4.2) widely observed children's development and provided an important push towards empirical research through the development of simple experimental tools that could be used to test **cognitive development** in children. Based on the findings, he developed a model with emerging landmarks of understanding taking place at specific times in childhood

(Piaget, 1959; Piaget and Inhelder, 1969). By the time we reach adolescence we've moved from initially sensory- and movement-oriented cognition, via mostly practice-based cognition, to highly systematic, logical and abstract thinking similar to that of adults.

Understanding of the **moral development** in childhood – what is right or wrong and why – was influenced considerably by the work of Lawrence Kohlberg (1984). He developed a series of moral dilemmas that he presented to children in different age groups. Based on their responses he identified how their perspective on what is good and bad is initially based on what feels good or bad, and what is rewarded and punished, after which the emphasis changes to what peers do, the rules at home and in school, laws they are subject to and, finally, more advanced thinking about social justice and ethics. Interestingly, research shows that while the overall trend of Kohlberg's theory is confirmed, even adults often use immature moral thinking and very few people tend to argue at the highest ethical level (Weiten, 2010). It is perhaps most relevant here for worried parents to understand that when young children are dishonest without feeling guilt it is because their morality is still primitive.

Freud's psychosexual stages have gone out of fashion, mainly perhaps because it is considered 'suspect' to consider children undergoing a sexual development before they are even ready to be sexually active. In particular, today's concerns around paedophilia and child pornography have contributed to this. For years Freud's perspectives dominated our perceptions and common terms like oral personality and anal personality (resulting from frustration in early childhood) have their origin in his work (Freud, 1940). If you are interested look it up.

Activity 4.2 *Active learning assignment*

Fact finding mission: look up videos online, discuss and answer the questions.

Jean Piaget	Renee Baillargeon
Describe the four stages in Piaget's model of cognitive development in children. Describe how children play in each stage. What are the main points of criticism of Piaget's model? What are the implications for nursing care for children?	Describe the study on object permanence conducted by Baillargeon with infants. How do her findings challenge Piaget's theories? How does her work make use of principles introduced by Robert Fantz? What are the implications for nursing care for infants?

Adolescence

Adolescence starts at different times for boys and girls (often earlier in girls) with considerable individual variations and it may span most of the teenage years. It is at this time that hormonal, intellectual and social developments prepare the person to cultivate an independent identity.

The development of personal **identity** was considered the core issue to resolve during this period according to Erikson (1959). James Marcia expanded this idea. In response to the identity crisis teenagers experience some seem to avoid the issue and show no concerns, which may attenuate maturity (identity diffusion); others seem to prematurely adopt or copy an identity pathway from others (identity foreclosure). Those who embrace the crisis may show an active struggle, trying on different roles and perspectives to postpone commitment to a particular identity (identity moratorium); which it is hoped will lead to successfully achieving a defined sense of identity (identity achievement) (Marcia, 1980). Because identity development is important, this is a period of great vulnerability. If there is a lack of close support and stability, teenagers may be in trouble. Children of divorced parents, ethnic minorities and gay and lesbian teenagers are sometimes at risk. The care for patients in adolescence should take into account that they can be highly sensitive to how their identity is perceived and recognised. Hormonal influences associated with puberty may also be an important issue that nurses need to find a way of coping with.

Case study: Obesity and identity

Jennifer is 15 years old. She is obese and newly diagnosed with Type 2 diabetes. She is in hospital because of her raised blood sugar level and she is quite ill. The aim of care is not only to stabilise Jennifer's diabetes, but also to educate her about her new medication regime and adopting a healthier lifestyle including weight loss and exercise. Jennifer is in a single room and at the moment she is refusing to have nurses come in to her unless absolutely essential. Her mother (who is also obese) stays with her all day. Although it is not in keeping with her dietary regime, Jennifer appears to be comfort eating by having takeaway fast food. Her mother says the hospital food is sub-standard and this is why she must feed her this way, at least sometimes. How would you analyse the problem? Think how, as a nurse, you might manage this situation to achieve the key goals of Jennifer's care. Write down your answers.

An outline response is provided at the end of the chapter.

Adulthood

Traditionally, **early adulthood** (20-35) is seen as the period in which physical abilities are maximised, studies are undertaken, professional careers are started, long term partnerships are formed and children appear on the scene. Parenthood means significant increases in responsibility and the need for maturity. Alternatively, if short-term or no partnerships prevail, significantly different life styles emerge. This is the stage that most nursing students are in. An age at which everything seems to be happening at the same time, the age of intense multi-tasking and juggling priorities. In case you have difficulty concentrating because there is something more important on your mind, it is not unthinkable that this is related to ... **love**! Yes, indeed you are in the age of love. While love is on our minds throughout our life span, this is the time when it is perhaps most closely related to what it is meant for: a very strong reminder that we are on this planet to reproduce.

Robert Sternberg seems to have understood this very well as he developed one of the few theories of love formulated within psychology. He suggested a triangular model consisting of three elements: **passion** (physical longing to initiate sex), **intimacy** (sharing and personal communication between partners) and **commitment** (the promise to stay together) (Sternberg, 1986). He theorised that a relationship that would last and could be successful when children would appear on the scene would need each of these three elements well represented in the relationship. The passion would ensure that a sexual relationship would be maintained. The intimacy is an essential binding factor – the 'glue' in the relationship, the core element in preventing conflict and alienation. The commitment would include the promise to put in a joint effort to raise offspring. He called this 'consummate love'. Cultures all over the world have formalised this in marriage vows. Sternberg included in his theory other types of love that might emerge if one of the factors was not there. For instance, he saw 'romantic love' as passion and intimacy without commitment. In Western culture many relationships start like this. In contrast, in other cultures, couples sometimes marry without really knowing each other, after an agreement between families. Such a marriage starts with only commitment ('empty love') and the hope that the two other elements develop over time. In many long-term relationships passion fades over time and couples end up with only intimacy and commitment or 'companionate love'. Although you may feel pity for these couples, research shows that many of them are not unhappy with such an arrangement (Sternberg, 1986). However, of course, it leaves the door ajar for a third person to come and provide the passion. The high divorce rate in many Western countries suggests that this scenario is far from theoretical.

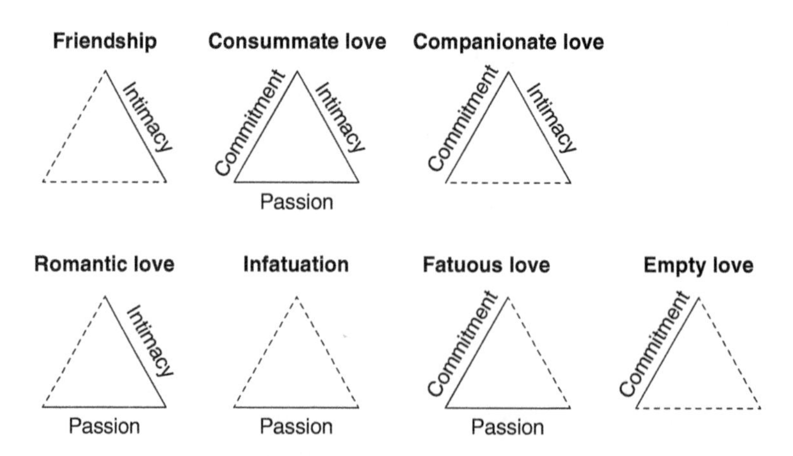

Figure 4.2: Seven types of love in Sternberg's triangular model of love

We are sure you will be able to imagine what the other types of love (see Figure 4.2) are like. The merits of Sternberg's model are its face validity (it makes sense) and the fact that it ties three aspects together that facilitate optimising having offspring and their survival through shared parental investment (Trivers, 1971). Another good thing is that the theory provides a way for couples to talk about their relationship in a more insightful way. As a nurse Sternberg's model may help you in establishing the quality of the partnerships of your patients, which will help predict their required levels of support.

Scenario: What's love got to do with it?

Aisha is a public health nurse who visits families in the neighbourhood. In a particularly problematic family it is evident that the parents are not communicating well with each other and that the passion has gone out of the relationship. This is reflected in extended conflicts and seems to trigger frequent misbehaviour in their four children. There are also several health problems in the family. How would you analyse the situation using Sternberg's triangular model of love? Discuss what a public health nurse could do to help.

An outline response is provided at the end of the chapter.

Middle adulthood (35–60) is often the time in which cognitive **maturity** and roles of leadership emerge. Experience and expertise become important assets and contribution to work and community flourish. Activities started in early adulthood often continue at a more intense pace, while physical abilities diminish. Hard work and stress are not unlikely to conspire and lead to stress-related illnesses in this period. A healthy life style in middle adulthood can prevent these calamities but, nonetheless, the average hospital would always have a significant number of people in this age group suffering with wear and tear or increased vulnerability related illnesses and a need for surgery (cardiovascular disease, cancer, diabetes etc.).

In **late adulthood (60+)** the traditional perspective is to emphasise decline and looking back on life. Retirement and the role of grandparent are particularly salient in this period, as is concern for legacy. Multiple health risks emerge and therefore most of your patients will be in this age group. Apart from health risks, it is important to realise that people remain fit longer and are living longer. The average life expectancy at birth in many rich countries has increased by 8–10 years since the 1960s. What has caused this is not easy to determine. Several factors seem to play a role: better medical care, less hard and unhealthy manual labour, better knowledge of health and fitness, better knowledge of environmental risk factors, a more active lifestyle. The extended life expectancy has brought about an important shift in outlook on ageing. The dominant perspective has evolved from an emphasis on disengagement from life as one is ageing (Cumming *et al.*, 1961) via activity promotion (Neugarten and Havighurst, 1969) to maintaining continuity in life (Atchley, 1980) and finding compensation for limitations (Baltes and Baltes, 1990). Most recently we are prone to accentuate the importance of maintaining a reciprocal relationship (giving as well as taking) with family and community (Wahrendorf *et al.*, 2010). As we see around us, it is not uncommon for someone to start entirely new activities in response to retirement. This often includes volunteer work in the community, arts, and fitness-related activities.

Successful ageing is a growing area of research with an increasing interest in what can make the autumn of our lives worthwhile. Cognitive fitness is perhaps the most essential of faculties to maintain a high quality of life. It is now evident that a broad scope of activities provides protection from the impact of ageing. The often used adage 'use it, or you'll lose it' is supported by research (Hultsch *et al.*, 1999; Swaab, 1991). An interesting experiment demonstrated that maintaining responsibility for a wide variety of physical and mental activities played an important role in maintaining both physical and mental fitness (Rodin and Langer, 1977). Nonetheless, rather sudden decline around 80 and particularly cognitive decline and dementia are still hard to predict and prevent. Even so, recent studies into Alzheimer's disease and its correlates has demonstrated that there are protective factors in continued and higher levels of education, engagement in change, and aerobic exercise (Erickson *et al.*, 2012).

Activity 4.3 — *Active learning assignment*

Fact finding mission: look up videos online, discuss, and answer the questions.

Erik Erikson	Ellen Langer
Describe the eight stages in Erikson's model of the life-span. How is personality affected by being successful/unsuccessful in each stage? What are the main points of criticism to Erikson's model? What are the implications for age-appropriate nursing care?	Describe Ellen Langer and collaborators' experimental studies on reversal of ageing in people in nursing homes. How does her work change perceptions of ageing? What are the implications for nursing care for older adults?

Learning

One of the reasons humans are so adaptable is because they have such a significant ability to learn. By learning we mean the **acquisition of new behaviours, emotions and understandings not based on maturation**. For people to develop into well-adjusted, effective and employable adults they need to learn a lot. Generally there is a recognition that we learn in at least four ways:

1. Association – classical conditioning (Pavlov, Watson), preparedness (Seligman).
2. Consequences – operant conditioning (Thorndike, Skinner).
3. Observation/imitation – modeling (Bandura).
4. Understanding – cognitive learning (Piaget).

Learning through association (including classical conditioning)

We are very good at remembering things that happened at the same time or in the same place. Babies learn to associate the mother's face with nurturing, her scent, and the sound of her voice. We learn words by their association with objects that are shown as the same time. We learn to associate our place of work, let's say a health-care organisation, with what happens there, what we do, and how it makes us feel. To make these associations we don't need to be aware and we don't need to understand. It just happens. In this way your patients will have learned to associate a hospital with their illness and the feelings associated with that. These feelings may come back when visiting a relative in hospital later. The longer they were in hospital and the more intense the experience, the stronger the association and the longer before this response fades out. Ivan Pavlov called this principle **classical conditioning** (see Chapter 2). While studying digestion in dogs he observed that they started salivating in response to a bell, metronome or light that coincided with the presentation of food (Pavlov, 1906). Once the dogs had started salivating on hearing the bell, this continued even when no food was given.

Watson demonstrated the same principle in humans. In an infamous experiment he conditioned a child (Little Albert) to become afraid of a white rat by producing a loud bang whenever the child was presented with the rat, of which it was initially not afraid at all (Watson and Rayner, 1920). Since then psychologists have been particularly interested in this mechanism as part of phobias. If you had a near-drowning experience, the lack of air triggers a panic reflex. The association of this experience with the presence of water will be strong and it is possible that your next encounter with water will produce the same panic response. While we have many other reflexes that can be conditioned, such as eye blinking, appetite, sexual excitement, and even a vague sense of discomfort, fear responses tend to be subject to rapid conditioning. Seligman (1971) demonstrated that classical conditioning of fear responses was much quicker if it involved an element that already had a natural potential to instil fear such as spiders, snakes, heights, water, or lightning. He called this 'preparedness'. Perhaps sharp objects such as injection needles also fall into this category.

Learning through association

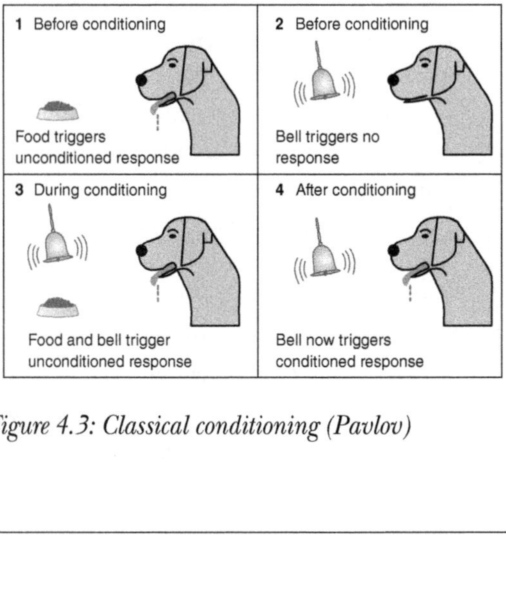

Figure 4.3: Classical conditioning (Pavlov)

Example in health care

Before you had experienced someone's heart stopping in the hospital a beep-beep-beep sound turning into a long beeeeeeeeeeeep at the bed side was not associated with fear. Once you experienced a cardiac arrest in the hospital accompanied by the change in beeps you learned to associate this sound with an emergency. Hearing it now generates the fear response you initially only felt when you responded to the cardiac arrest itself. Even alarm clocks that produce this kind of sound might generate a fear response in you.

Learning from consequences (operant learning or conditioning)

We also learn from the consequences of our behaviour. Thorndike's law of effect states it as follows: 'responses that produce a satisfying effect in a particular situation become more likely to occur again in that situation, and responses that produce a discomforting effect become less likely to occur again in that situation' (Thorndike, 1927). We use the term **operant conditioning** for this learning mechanism. We learn to repeat behaviour that is rewarded (reinforced), and may not do so with behaviour that is punished. In humans many different things can be conceived as reward or punishment or discouragement. Eventually it is the impact of events on pleasure or pain centres in the brain that determines whether we experience something as rewarded or punished. It is important to realise that we are highly sensitive in this department. For instance, very subtle facial signals can be received as 'reinforcement' (smile) or discouragement (raised eyebrows). Skinner believed that virtually all of human behaviour is essentially shaped in this way (Skinner, 1972). His research with animals provided a host of new insights into the extent of the impact of this type of learning. For instance, he found that instant rewards are more effective than ones given later. This is why we find it so difficult to stop unhealthy behaviours which give us initial pleasure, and so hard to learn healthy behaviours that only have long-term benefits and initial aversive effects, such as giving up smoking or drinking. Incidentally, the ability to suppress the urge for immediate reinforcement seemed to predict success in life. In a famous longitudinal study, researchers gave children the opportunity to eat a marshmallow or to wait and receive a second one. Those that could wait turned out to have better jobs and earn more money later in life (Mischel and Moore, 1973).

Learning from consequences

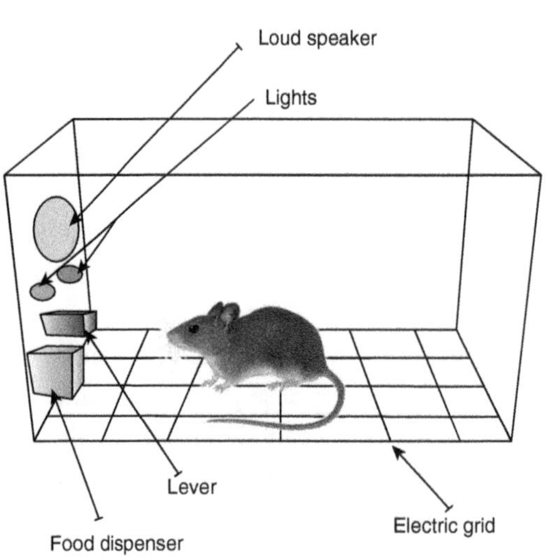

Figure 4.4: Operant conditioning: the Skinner box

Example in health care

When you first explain surgery procedures to a patient you may be unsure how to do it. Patients may be more scared after you talk with them. Every time this happens you may tell yourself 'not this way'. You feel punished. When it works well and your patients smile or tell you that your explanations make them feel better, you feel rewarded. You tell yourself, this is the way to do it. Gradually the reinforcement of the right way and the discouragement of the wrong way will help shape a proficient way of giving information.

Learning through observation/imitation (modelling or observational learning)

Although much of mammal learning is the result of operant and classical conditioning, complex sequences of behaviour that could, theoretically perhaps, be learned through shaping (operant conditioning) tend to be acquired faster, more effectively and more safely through **modelling or observational learning**. It is much better for a fox to learn how to hunt from an experienced mother than to embark on a perilous process of trial and error in which the punishment for the wrong move may be instant death. It is the same for us. Our children learn how to use electrical appliances, knives and scissors from observing a parent's safe demonstration. It is evident that not only positive but also negative behaviour may be subject to modelling. Seminal research on modelling in children was done by Albert Bandura who demonstrated that seeing a film of adult aggressive behaviour with a big inflatable doll (Bobo Doll study) led to aggressive play by children when they were allowed in a room that contained the doll. Children who had not seen the film did not play aggressively with the doll (Bandura *et al.*, 1963).

Learning through imitation	Example in health care
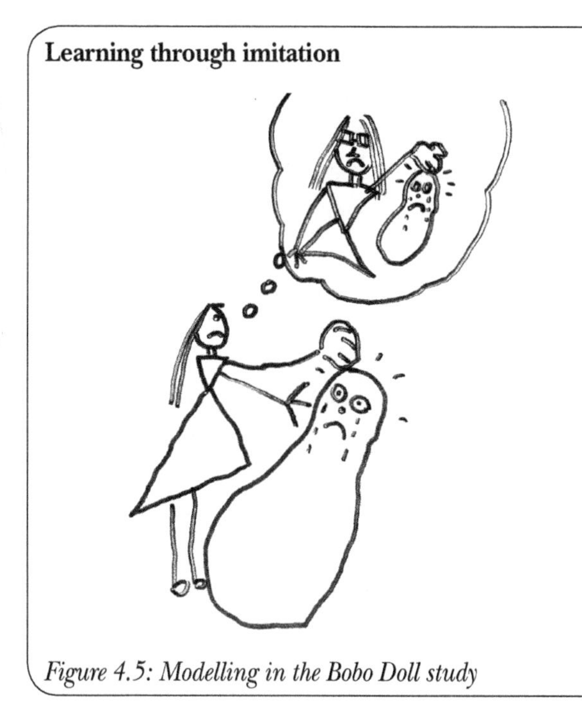 *Figure 4.5: Modelling in the Bobo Doll study*	When you started your first placement you were not sure how to greet new patients in an appropriate way, how to find out a bit about their background, and how to establish a friendly relationship. Fortunately, your preceptor had a very good way of doing this. You observed the behaviour and practised modelling after it until you started to get it right yourself.

Nurses will learn a lot from observing experienced nurses. In particular, performance on complex technical nursing tasks, such as intubation, giving injections, wound dressing etc. benefits considerably from the inclusion of demonstrations by proficient models.

Learning by understanding (cognitive learning)

While the first three types of learning do not seem to require conscious reflection it would seem that this aspect is at the core of how we learn highly complex, theoretical and abstract material. In simple terms, anything that requires understanding falls under **cognitive learning**. Piaget (Piaget, 1976) suggested that conceptual learning starts very early in life and is the result of two core processes, **assimilation** and **accommodation**. When developing a conceptual understanding, children try to fit much of their reality into it. For instance, the word 'mamma' may be used for the mother, but other women are also assimilated into the concept which, for a while, seems to include all women. Of course, when the infant is corrected on this it will have to change or 'accommodate' its conceptual understanding to 'mamma is only one person'. We do the same with other concepts and even as you are reading this book you are alternately using the two processes to enhance your conceptual mastery of the complexities of this world. Assimilation tends to feel pleasant, integrates, and seems to confirm you are thinking in the right way, whereas accommodation provides a challenge because it comes with the need for an adjustment effort, which we don't always like. Overall, all learning that includes understanding, thinking or complex processing of information falls under cognitive learning. We'll come back to this when we address cognition in more detail (Chapter 6).

Learning by understanding	**Example in health care**
Jean Piaget and Cognitive Development: Assimilation and Accommodation How can a young girl use her 'dog schema' when encountering a cat? • She can **assimilate** the experience into her schema by referring to the cat as a 'dog' or • She can **accommodate** her animal schema by separating the cat, and even different types of dogs, into separate schemas.	When you first arrived in the hospital you communicated in the same way with all patients. You assimilated all patients into one way of understanding them. After a while you learned that some patients felt confident communicating with you, while others were reticent. You learned to accommodate your communication into a different manner for open and reticent patients. For a while you assimilated all patient communication into either one or the other approach. Later you learned to accommodate your concept of communication with patients further to respond effectively to diverse individuals.

Scenario: Awareness of conditioning and learning

Identify principles of learning in this scenario.

Charles is a nursing student who has observed a phlebotomist who was extracting blood samples from children. He was not looking forward to it but, to his surprise, the phlebotomist met almost no resistance from children and almost none cried. Later in the day the phlebotomist explains her way of working.

- *A child-friendly environment is generated and (mobiles, posters, toys) are used to distract children from the blood test.*
- *Warming up the palm or arm is used as a distraction for the nerves, which will react to the warmth and thus experience less pain.*

continued . . .

continued . . .

- *A quick skilled overall assessment of child and parent, and their anxiety level, determines the level of distraction needed. For some this might be simply looking at the pictures on the wall, for others it may take a few moments of play beforehand, possibly with a mock needle and teddy.*
- *The phlebotomist is also aware of the child's past medical history, experience and understanding of blood tests.*
- *Localised analgesia cream is used as pain relief on the hand or arm.*

An outline response is provided at the end of the chapter.

Learning is often a complex (and messy) process

Very often the different types of learning interact and may happen at the same time. It is possible that different types of learning operate at the same time or build on one another. You may, for instance, learn how to compute quantities of medication by understanding the formulas you use (cognitive learning), but also from observing an experienced nurse who shows you how it is done in practice and by imitating this nurse's method (modelling). Once you start doing it yourself you perfect the skill by learning from your mistakes and successes (operant conditioning). It is possible that one type of learning interferes with the other. An exasperated preceptor famously said to a student nurse: 'Now shut up, I don't want to hear another word. You need to learn to listen'. Evidently, the preceptor tried to discourage behaviour she perceived as lacking listening ability. However, at the same time, she modelled lack of listening ability herself to the student. A parent who severely punishes a child for beating up a younger sibling makes the same mistake. It is also possible that instructions (cognitive learning) and a demonstration (modelling) show discrepancies. Another complicating element is that there is often overlap between the two types of conditioning. Phobias tend to be learned through classical conditioning, but the punishing character of the anxiety also suggests that operant conditioning is involved. Please embrace this complexity in Activity 4.4. It should be enlightening!

Activity 4.4 *Decision making*

Analyse these examples and determine whether and in what way each way of learning might be involved.

	Association (Classical conditioning)	Consequences (Operant conditioning)	Observation & Imitation (Modelling)	Understanding (Cognitive learning)
Giving an injection				
Taking blood pressure				
Fear of blood				

continued . . .

continued . . .

	Association (Classical conditioning)	Consequences (Operant conditioning)	Observation & Imitation (Modelling)	Understanding (Cognitive learning)
How to reassure patients				
Communicate effectively				
White coat phobia				

An outline answer is provided at the end of the chapter.

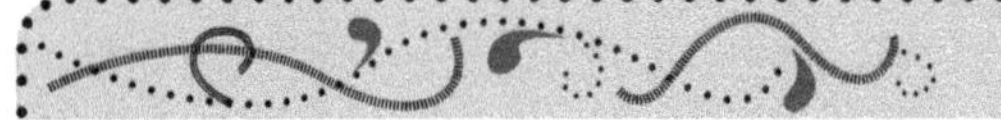

Chapter summary

- The interaction between nature and nurture is complex and it is essential to realise that they always interact. Nature will not express itself without nurture and, in turn, nurture is affected by nature. Children affect their development actively rather than being passive recipients of parenting and education.
- Spring in the Brain is the process whereby stimulation in an enriched environment prepares a child neurologically for life in a complex world. Deprivation in this period could do irreparable damage to a child's future.
- Stage theories provide a useful blueprint of how people in the Western world develop during the life span. It is important not to take the stages too literally.
- While four mechanisms of learning have been identified, the reality is that these mechanisms interact in complex ways.
- Nurses who understand developmental and learning mechanisms and are able to translate these into their care practice will be more effective and more sensitive in their dealings with patients and colleagues. They will also have a better understanding of themselves and their functioning as nurses.

Activities: brief outline answers

Case study: Developmental deprivation in hospital (see page 58)

Neural development (Spring in the Brain) may be compromised in a hospital due to lack of stimulation, activity, individual and active play. It is essential for nurses to do what is possible to compensate. Fortunately, nowadays, 24-hour visiting by parents is facilitated, encouraged and recommended in many countries of the world including the UK. Whenever possible, care at home would be preferable in Christopher's case.

Case study: Attachment (see page 60)

It is very common in NICU to encourage and facilitate mother and child bonding including close skin-to-skin contact, eye contact and generally spending time together. If breast feeding is possible it should be facilitated. Overall this period of a baby's life is crucial to its personal development and the development of the attachment with its mother. Although priority is given to physical and physiological needs, as babies' conditions in NICU are often life threatening, close attention should be given to parent-child bonding at this important life stage. It is important to take the parent's vulnerability just after birth into account.

Case study: Attention deficit and hyperactivity disorder (ADHD) (see page 61)

Clearly the social worker on the team may become involved in terms of assessing child safety. Perhaps his mother would benefit from a parenting course. This would help her understand the various types of parenting and perhaps reflect on her own style. Such courses are often delivered in groups and she may receive help and support from other parents who are coping with similar difficulties. The acquired skills may benefit the child's ADHD behaviours. Overall, rewarding good behaviour rather than punishing poor behaviour needs to be encouraged. His mother might also benefit from one-to-one counselling as dealing with ADHD can be very challenging and stressful.

Case study: Obesity and identity (see page 63)

Family dynamics evidently play a key role in Jennifer's obesity. Therefore, health promotion efforts need to involve the whole family. You are bound to encounter resistance and teenage rebelliousness may be a hindrance. Simply telling either Jennifer or her mother what to do is reminiscent of the authoritarian parental model, and therefore may only have limited success. It might even be destructive for both the relationship and Jennifer's ongoing learning about diabetes. Therefore, developing a good relationship with Jennifer and her mother is essential to conquering this (this also applies to the dietician). The NMC (2010, p. 24) informs us that 'all nurses must use excellent communication and interpersonal skills' and it is using these skills that will be pivotal. Remember that while Jennifer is still in hospital you can still influence the situation.

Scenario: What's love got to do with it? (see page 65)

Evidently lack of passion and intimacy in the relationship qualifies as 'empty love' in Sternberg's model. The resulting lack of coherence in the family may be the cause or a compounding factor in all problems. Trying to address the children's behavioural issues and health problems in isolation without including the relationship between the parents would be a mistake. This would be a matter for discussion in the multi-disciplinary team (MDT). Aisha might be in a position to start the parents thinking about how their relationship might affect the sense of security within the family and how that affects the health and behaviour of the children.

Scenario: Awareness of conditioning and learning (see page 70)

The phlebotomist has developed a method that reduces the chance that the children she is taking blood from develop anxiety through classical and operant conditioning; she provides a good model for Charles and, by explaining how she works, she allows Charles to also strengthen his cognitive learning in the area of giving injections.

Activity 4.4: Decision making (see page 71)

Giving an injection is learned first and foremost by modelling by an experienced nurse and understanding principles and precise instructions (cognitive); shaping may play a role in refining the skill based on encouraging and discouraging reactions from patients.

Taking blood pressure is learned like giving an injection; because there is less risk of hurting patients the shaping process may follow the other instructions sooner.

Fear of blood is learned through classical conditioning and possibly maintained through operant conditioning; by avoiding situations in which you might see blood you keep your fear of blood low; this reinforces the avoidance and cements the phobia.

How to reassure patients – good modelling will be really helpful, but understanding of how best to do this is essential; shaping the skill will take place by operant learning.

Communicate effectively: such as by reassuring patients.

White coat phobia is acquired by patients through classical conditioning, perhaps in early childhood; by avoiding doctor's visits this anxiety can be kept low; this reinforces the avoidance and thus the phobia can intensify; patients suffering from white coat phobia might read about the dangers of the medical profession to support their anxiety (cognitive).

Further reading

DeHart, G., Sroufe, A. L. and Cooper R. G. (2005) *Child development: Its nature and course* (5th Ed.). Boston, MA: McGraw-Hill.

There are many good introductions to child development, but this one is particularly accessible.

Sroufe, L. A. (2005) Attachment and development: a prospective, longitudinal study from birth to adulthood. *Attachment & human development*, 7(4): 349–367.

This article explores the impact of attachment over time. This journal is worth exploring.

Kail, R. and Cavanaugh, J. (2015) *Human development: a life-span view* (7th Ed.). Belmont (CA): Cengage Learning.

This recent text covers changing perspectives on the life span very well. Earlier editions can be accessed online.

Useful websites

http://www.learner.org/resources/series138.html

The famous Discovering Psychology series hosted by Prof. Philip Zimbardo, watch number 5: The Developing Child.

https://en.wikipedia.org/wiki/Nature_versus_nurture

Wikipedia's entry on the nature<>nurture debate provides significant background.

http://listverse.com/2008/03/07/10-modern-cases-of-feral-children/

Contemporary cases of feral children illustrate the importance of early child development.

https://www.youtube.com/watch?v=Mt4N9GSBoMI

Here is a YouTube video illustrating Operant Conditioning in the *Big Bang Theory* television series. YouTube has many relevant videos. Use keywords such as: Skinner – operant conditioning, Pavlov – classical conditioning, Bandura – Bobo Doll or Piaget.

Chapter 5
Consciousness and memory

Chapter aims

After reading this chapter you will be able to:

- describe how awareness and consciousness are essential to our functioning and why we can only focus on a limited number of items at the same time;
- understand how different activities require different levels of consciousness and why we are not conscious of all our activities;
- understand the dynamics of sleep and its impact on wellbeing with a view to recognising effective and ineffective sleep in yourself and people in your care;
- explain how your memory works and how you can improve it in your nursing practice;
- provide examples of the limitations of your memory and how it can be unreliable.

Consciousness and memory are addressed in one chapter because they work together to allow us to act with intention and to integrate our experiences in daily activities, thinking and decision making. The section on consciousness is important because fluctuations in levels of consciousness in yourself and your patients are frequent and need to be understood. We also discuss the unconscious aspect of our functioning, the dynamics of sleep, and how good quality sleep is essential for the wellbeing of humans generally, and particularly for the patients in your care. We look at the mechanisms of memory and its strengths and limitations, which is important in nursing. Both consciousness and memory have clear limitations so you must not be too confident and always check when you have to rely on your awareness or memory for important tasks. We also address how we can make effective use of memory within the health-care setting.

Consciousness

Consciousness is usually defined as 'a person's perceptions, thoughts, and feelings at any given moment' (p. 199) or 'an individual's current awareness of external and internal stimuli' (p. 197) (Nolen-Hoeksema *et al.*, 2014). Consciousness helps us to monitor our surroundings and our own information processing. This facilitates making choices, solving problems, planning and controlling our behaviour. Consciousness is part of the perceptual process, thinking, attention and awareness. As we indicated in Chapter 2, philosophers and psychologists have long been fascinated with consciousness. Has this helped us uncover all of its mysteries? The answer is 'no'. Daniel Dennett, one of the foremost thinkers on this issue considers 'consciousness systematically outside of science' (Cohen and Dennett, 2011, p. 363). Even the boldest neuroscientists tend to be cautious in their explanations of consciousness (Laureys and Tononi, 2011). They suspect consciousness in many parts of the brain (Damasio *et al.*, 2009) and many emphasise the importance of the reticular formation in the hindbrain and midbrain, which activates attention in the cerebral cortex (Damasio *et al.*, 2009). Another avenue of enquiry is into so-called 'mirror-neurons' that seem to allow us to monitor our own processing (Stamenov and Gallese, 2002). This suggests that consciousness is an attentional process that allows awareness and reflection on what we do, feel, or think.

Concept summary: Consciousness, memory, worry, and living in the moment.

When you are worried, helpful friends sometimes utter the wonderful phrase, 'You should learn to live more in the moment'. However, this is easier said than done. In fact, it goes against human nature. Human consciousness includes regurgitating the past and worrying about the future. As hunter-gatherers we needed to remember our past experiences to learn from them and then to project that learning into expectations for the future to stand a chance of survival. Fortunately, we have phenomenal memories. We have the amazing ability to consciously recall, re-experience and use memories to imagine our future. This allows us to adapt, survive, and make sense of our lives. Humans with high conscious awareness and good memories will have survived in larger numbers than those without these qualities. It may also be true that the survival rate of humans prone to worry surpassed that of those who 'only lived in the moment'. In its most absolute form, living entirely in the moment is the horror of dementia. The moment our memory stops registering what just happened, life becomes rather meaningless.

Levels of consciousness

Generally, we would consider inanimate objects such as stones as not conscious. Also in plants we do not assume any level of consciousness. In many animals, particularly in mammals, it is evident that they are conscious, but are their conscious abilities the same as ours? Perhaps not. Dennett identified four levels of consciousness (see Table 5.1.) related to the degree of intention in our behaviour or thinking (Dennett, 1993). At its lowest level, and similar to all mammals, humans exhibit reflexes that take place without being conscious of them, although we may become conscious of them afterwards, (think of knee jerks, eye blinks and sudden scares). At a second level we are aware of a goal to be achieved (you are hungry, thirsty, bored). At a third level we are also aware of the means to reach the goal (you are hungry so you think about what you would like to eat and are on your way to the fridge). Up to this level many animals would match us; however, they may not generally achieve the fourth and highest level at which we reflect on ourselves and are conscious of how events are perceived by others (what will others think of me when they hear me rummage in the fridge in the middle of the night?). This requires observing oneself and imagining other people's intentions and states of mind. For nurses it is essential to be able to operate at this level to provide high quality care. Nurses need to be able to reflect, put themselves in the position of the patient and understand their feelings, thoughts and behaviours. Only in this way can their comfort and dignity be maintained (Walsh and Kowanko, 2002). Likewise, the nurse needs to be conscious of his or her own motives, feelings, thoughts and behaviours. If we look at it like this, it would seem essential that nurses become highly conscious and reflective practitioners (we'll come back to this in Chapter 6 and Chapter 10); see Mindfulness (Langer and Moldoveanu, 2000).

Table 5.1: Levels of consciousness

Levels of consciousness	Examples in nursing
1. Reflexes (not conscious)	You recoil when seeing an ugly wound; startle when you hear a loud noise; smile when something funny happens; jump to assist a patient who almost has a fall.
2. Needs, drives, goals (low consciousness)	You realise you are hungry, thirsty, in need of a good night's sleep, or something to lift your mood; you are aware of a patient who needs help.
3. Strategies (medium consciousness)	Computing a daily medication dose for a patient; developing a treatment plan; deciding what to do to reduce a patient's fever; listen well, show empathy.
4. Reflection, taking another's perspective (high consciousness)	Reflection on your care after you've just completed a care activity with a patient; reflection on how a patient might have taken 'bad news' about unsuccessful treatment.

The 'camera analogy' of consciousness (MacLennan, 1996; Jaynes, 2000)

As you are reading this, your focus, your awareness, your consciousness is with the words you are reading and the page they are written on. While you are reading you also become aware of the thoughts you have about what you are reading. It almost seems like there is a camera that points towards the book in the outside world and then shifts to how you make sense of its content in your head. Thus we go back and forth really quickly, so quickly that you seem to attend to both external and internal elements at the same time. You may sense this shift best when you are lost in thought and suddenly an urgent event outside you requires your full attention. Conversely, an important thought may suddenly pop into your head and it draws your attention away from the outside world. Funnily enough, we don't always sense that we are interrupting our activities when this shifting back and forth happens during 'multi-tasking'. As we will see in the next section, shifts in focus in our awareness may not be as absolute as the camera metaphor suggests.

Scenario: Consciousness and distraction

Sue talks with a patient about the treatment plan. While she is listening, several diagnostic and treatment-related thoughts are formed. She shifts back and forth between these thoughts and paying direct attention to the patient. It requires effort and concentration but she realises that she needs both types of awareness in this situation. In the middle of it all she suddenly realises she forgot her mother's birthday yesterday. Her forgetfulness upsets her and her concentration on the patient is gone. How can she restore her focus?

An outline response is provided at the end of the chapter.

The unconscious

Essential for the understanding of consciousness is that we are not continuously aware of all of our activities and that consciousness is limited. In fact, much of our processing eludes consciousness entirely or takes place at lower levels. Some of our 'unconscious' is of a purely physical nature, such as digestive activities, internal muscle coordination, the processing needed to keep heart and circulation going, etc. There is a reason why we are not conscious of these functions. This way we can't mess them up. However, there are also complex activities that we are aware of when we are learning them, but that become automatic once we've mastered them. At this point we are no longer conscious of how we perform them. Once well-learned, we can drive a car while listening and talking to a companion, without being conscious of driving-related processing.

Case study: Consciousness and experience

Sam is an experienced nurse who takes blood pressure while talking with patients. This is much appreciated. Of course, a conversation cannot be had without being conscious of it, but much of the physical activity associated with measuring blood pressure has become automatic and can be performed without being conscious of every step. You ask Sam about it and he tells you that this is the result of years of experience. 'Don't be fooled though, there are moments when I am just focusing on the task at hand, and will only return to the conversation when I am confident that I have a correct reading. Also, when I have to think deeply about what the patient says, I have to stop what I am doing.' How could you emulate Sam, even if you are not as experienced?

An outline response is provided at the end of the chapter.

Freud (1922) considered that the understanding of our unconscious operations is essential to make sense of what is really on our minds, especially when we are struggling with our mental health. He introduced the idea that we tend to 'repress' internal conflicts, strong urges we cannot satisfy, or memories of traumatic experiences to the extent that we are no longer aware of them. Repression is an involuntary mechanism that leads to hiding or making inaccessible such elements from consciousness. They might only find expression in dreams, automatic associations, or slips of the tongue (Freud and Brill, 1916). Contemporary sources highlight something similar called **dissociation**. Dissociation or numbing is most often described as the uncoupling of the emotional aspect from our experience, which can occur after very intense fear during a traumatic experience (Van der Kolk and McFarlane, 2012; Van der Kolk *et al.*, 1996). After emotional centres (mainly amygdala) get overwhelmed during the ordeal of a traumatic event, they become desensitised and subsequently cease to produce intense emotions. This is a neurological phenomenon that is essentially a protective adaptation because it helps us to cope with further potentially life-threatening events. However, after normality has resumed, persistent dissociation can be highly debilitating. Without felt emotions we cannot function very well. We find it hard to relate to other people and make decisions because we no longer 'feel' what the right choice is. When suffering from dissociation, life can become very bland and meaningless, like eating without tasting the food. People lose the 'appetite for life'.

The unconscious patient

You will encounter patients who are in various states of diminished consciousness (Figure 5.1) (disorientation, obtund, lethargy, stupor, coma), often as a result of accidents, cardiac arrest, stroke, poisoning, chemical deficits, etc. Sometimes unconsciousness is induced by medics to protect the patient. Many operations require a full anaesthetic, which reduces activity in the brain with the purpose of preventing the conscious experience of the operation. This is closely monitored before and during the operation. Therefore, most patients wake up afterwards with no recollection of the experience and the pain they might otherwise have endured. On rare occasions (0.1–1 per cent of operations) the patient wakes up during the operation, which can be traumatic (Akkerman and Knape, 2014). Overall, patients tend to be most fearful of the

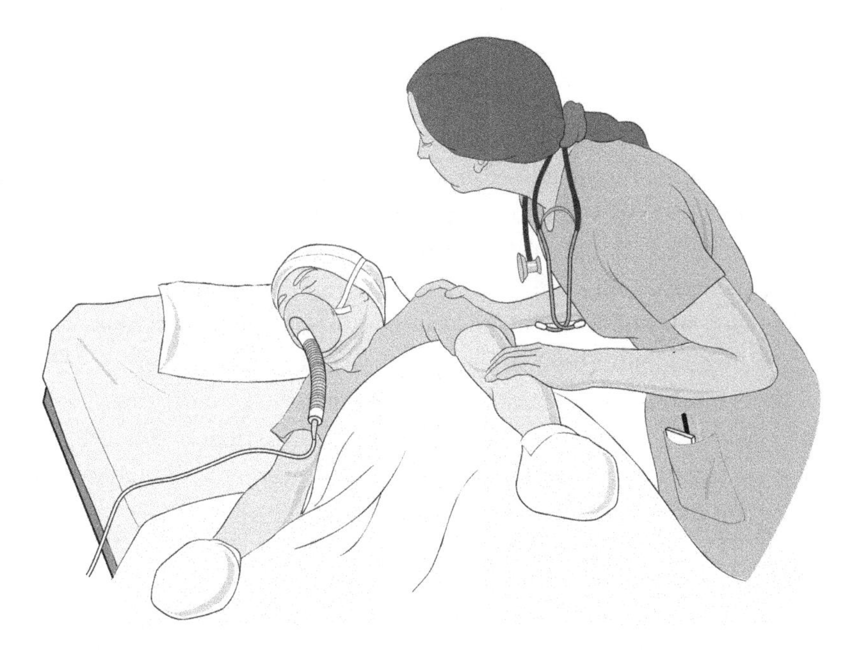

Figure 5.1: The unconscious patient

general anaesthetic because of possible post-operative pain or not waking up afterwards (Mavridou *et al.*, 2013). To wilfully give up one's consciousness requires trust on the part of the patient, and the nurse plays an important role in instilling this trust.

Activity 5.1 *Critical thinking*

In what way are people in these conditions conscious (or not)? (Refer to Table 5.1.)

Condition	
A nurse who is multi-tasking.	
A patient under full anaesthetic.	
A nurse who is performing routine activities in a rush.	
A person with a profound intellectual disability (PIMD) who cannot communicate with or respond to care givers.	
A man in a coma.	
A woman affected by locked-in syndrome.	
Someone meditating or praying.	
A girl affected by mind altering drugs at a dance party.	
A neonate just before and after birth.	
An older adult affected by severe dementia.	

An outline answer is provided at the end of the chapter.

Altered consciousness

While we may be fearful of losing consciousness, altering it has been of significant interest throughout human history. Knowledge of fermentation processes, and therefore the ability to manufacture alcoholic beverages, goes back thousands of years. There is pre-historic evidence of festivities that have included drinking alcohol to disinhibit those participating. Smoking (tobacco, cannabis, opium) or eating mind-altering substances (mushrooms) also have a long history, often in combination with rituals and shamanistic activities. Most major religious texts mention the use of fasting, meditation without sleep, and sensory deprivation (retreating into a cave or the desert) to induce states of exaltation and hallucinations in order to alter consciousness in such a way as to become receptive to religious or spiritual experiences. Such experiences were considered of great significance. To this day, prolonged prayer and meditation sessions are an important part of spiritual expansion of consciousness.

Altered and altering consciousness in health care

In hospitals we encounter the impact of excessive use of mind-altering substances on individuals as they present with effects of misuse of alcohol, cigarettes, heroin, cocaine and other recreational drugs. We also encounter the direct effects and side-effects of anaesthetics, pain relief, sleeping tablets, and a wide variety of other substances that alter consciousness in the patient. With psychoactive drugs, drugs that affect our brain, we discriminate between **stimulants** (which heighten neural connectivity) and **depressants** (which reduce connectivity). In particular, stimulants may lead to dramatic changes in how we perceive the world and ourselves. Too much of any of these substances can be very dangerous and even lead to death. Because of this it is gradually becoming more common to use non-pharmacological interventions where possible. In particular, to induce sleep or for pain and anxiety reduction (see Chapter 9) there are methods such as relaxation and distraction techniques, yoga, or meditation. These can bring about considerable reductions in sympathetic activation and change consciousness. They may also play a role in palliative care. Hypnosis can be used as a tool to reduce focus on pain or anxiety and induce relaxation. The idea of hypnosis in health care is to submit to suggestions from a hypnotist regarding behaviours you would like to change but for which you think you lack the strength of will.

We also come across the need to boost consciousness and instil new liveliness in patients who have been hospitalised. Long-term admissions and chronic conditions, especially in geriatric care, can turn active and able people into passive, dependent and helpless patients. To reactivate those affected in this way is an important task for nurses. The return of responsibilities, choice, communication, aerobic exercise and challenging activities is most likely to bring about higher levels of functioning and consciousness (Rodin and Langer, 1977).

Case study: Overcoming helplessness

Mary is 72 years old and was admitted to the cardiac care unit (CCU) following a myocardial infarction (MI). After a couple of weeks, the nurse in charge is discussing her medication management and home discharge. Her prognosis is very good. Indeed, with gradual restoration to activity she should be able to regain her independence and have a good quality of life. Unfortunately, Mary is rather disoriented and has been strongly affected by the weeks of inactivity. Furthermore she seems to have accepted her present incapacity and temporary wheelchair use within the hospital as a permanent feature of her life. What can a nurse do to address this problem?

An outline response is provided at the end of the chapter.

Sleep

Many nurses will spend a lot of time around sleeping people. So it is important to understand how sleep works. Sleeping is not the same as being unconscious. We've known this for a long time because during sleep we dream and we tend to be aware of dreams while we have them and afterwards when we wake up. More recently, research with the electroencephalograph (EEG) has demonstrated that neural activity when asleep is different from wakefulness and varies considerably during an average night's sleep (see Figure 5.2). Much of the research on sleep was done in so called sleep labs (Edinger *et al.*, 2004). Participants in such studies typically volunteered to sleep over in the researcher's lab and were connected to EEG instruments measuring neural activity in the brain. What we learned from the research is that during an average night we go back and forth between different types of sleep (see Figure 5.2), from more shallow to deep sleep, which could be identified by distinctly different patterns of brainwaves. Shallow sleep was also identified as the type of sleep in which **rapid eye movements (REM)** occurred and most dreams were reported if participants were awoken. The deepest sleep was less eventful with neural brainwaves suggesting mostly activity limited to breathing, heartbeat and metabolism. There are a few transitional stages between REM and deep sleep that could also be identified on the basis of EEG findings (stages 1–3). The deepest sleep (stage 4) tends to occur mostly in the first half of the night. REM sleep, while present for brief periods in the first four hours, is more dominant in the second half of the night. We tend to be very still during REM sleep, but may move around in the bed in the other stages. It is thought that deep sleep helps us recover from physical exertion, while REM sleep deals with recovery from mental fatigue and stress. This explains why you might wake up after four hours feeling physically but not mentally rested. It is evident that we need REM sleep as much as deep sleep and if we don't get enough of it we start experiencing dreamlike episodes and hallucinations while we are awake. If you wake up patients who were in deep sleep, they may be more disoriented than when they were in REM sleep.

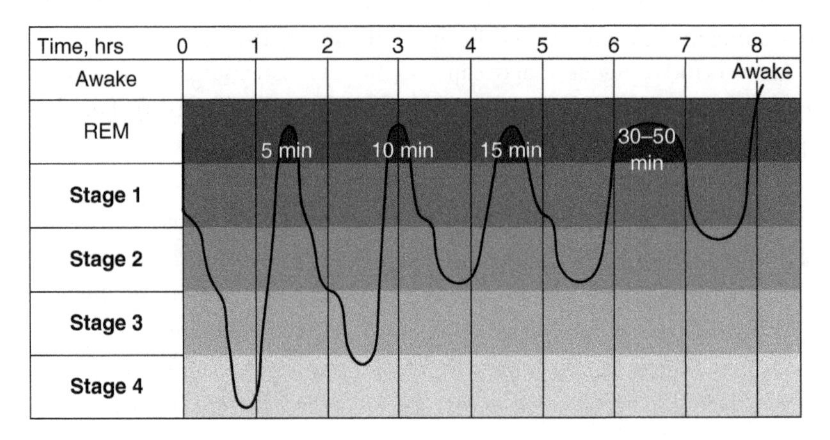

Figure 5.2: Average sleep pattern in adults

Sleep patterns evolve during the life span. Babies sleep many times during the day. Small children need an afternoon sleep in addition to a good night's sleep, while adolescents tend to sleep for about nine hours. Adults in Britain sleep just over seven hours on average (Bin *et al.*, 2012). In late adulthood sleep can be negatively affected by low levels of melatonin in the brain, which makes going to sleep difficult or leads to frequent disruptions of sleep. It is safe to say that good sleep is essential to be energetic and physically and mentally healthy. Sleep patterns can be disrupted by nightmares, sleepwalking, sleep talking, night terrors, sleep apnoea and snoring. Some drugs and alcohol specifically suppress REM sleep. Sleeping pills may provide a temporary solution when patients can't sleep, but need to be used with caution because, in the long run, they can disrupt sleep patterns even more.

Research summary

- Sleep disturbances in hospitals are common (Bernhofer *et al.*, 2014), in particular after surgery (Orr and Stahl, 1977) or traumatic brain injury (Ponsford *et al.*, 2013). Study of sleep disturbances in geriatric hospitals (night-time insomnia, daytime sleepiness and sleep-onset delay) predicted significantly higher mortality rates at follow-up after two years (Manabe *et al.*, 2000).
- Nightshifts and long working hours may affect sleep in nurses, which creates fatigue, which, in turn, is an important risk factor for the occurrence of workplace accidents and mistakes (Smith-Miller *et al.*, 2014). However, a recent scoping review of the impact of 12-hour shifts did not demonstrate evidence of the impact of the length of the shift on patient outcomes (Harris *et al.*, 2015). Maintaining regularity in a nurse's sleeping patterns, as much as possible, preserves sleep quality and prevents insomnia and day-time fatigue (Chou *et al.*, 2015).

Dreams

Why we dream is a source of dispute among psychologists. Some would say that we dream to solve problems (Cartwright, 1974). Others emphasise dreams as ways of wish fulfilment (Freud, 2010. First published in 1899). Much has been written about symbolism and hidden meanings in dreams, but many researchers today suggest that dreams might just be meaningless imagery strung together and triggered by haphazard brain activation (McCarley and Hobson, 1979). This does not have to mean that dreams are without purpose. For instance, why would trauma victims often have nightmares in which they relive traumatic events they experienced (Littlewood *et al.*, 2015)?

Scenario: How have you slept?

When Consuela is asking her patients in the morning, 'How have you slept?' she is potentially doing much more than making conversation. She gets information on the overall sleep satisfaction as an indicator of wellbeing. Also, she may get an idea whether enough deep sleep and REM sleep was achieved. If patients report nightmares she probes to learn more because if this is recurring problem and traumatic or fear-provoking imagery occurs, this may be an indicator of a stress response. Consuela also checks if the patient's sleep may be affected by medication and day-time naps. What would you suggest can be done to optimise sleep in patients in general?

An outline response is provided at the end of the chapter.

Memory

From consciousness to memory is not a big step because they operate in intertwined ways. Without memory we can't be conscious of our past and consciousness helps us memorise new experiences. Memory is important and we feel blessed if we consider ourselves to have a good memory. Just like with consciousness, there is a lot that we do not know about memory and what we do know we have learned quite recently.

Memory and the brain

It stands to reason that the neural events and circuitry involved in any experience might somehow be involved to recall it later on. When we experience something, neurons send messages to different parts of the brain to process the information. Action potentials and synaptic transmission from one neuron to another generate this process. The pattern of neural activation somehow represents the event. The **consolidation** of these patterns of transmission in the form of chemical and structural changes in synapses and the growth of new dendrites generates a possibility to more or less repeat these patterns later on during recall. It is thought that this process takes place all over the brain, but that the hippocampal area (sub-cortical) plays a specific role in generating this process of consolidation, as well as the integrated recall of events. Consolidation is also referred to as long-term potentiation (LTP) or a long-lasting increase in neural responsiveness in synapses (Ward, 2010). Some of this may happen fast and directly in the neurons, whereas other forms of consolidation occur more slowly and involve the hippocampus. The more a memory has been consolidated, the more likely it will be that you can spontaneously recall it. Without consolidation only recognition may be possible.

Integrated memory model

Before we had empirical knowledge of the neuroscience of memory, there were theoretical efforts to describe and organise prevailing perspectives on how memory works. The multi-store or modal model (Atkinson and Shiffrin, 1968) is still considered a more or less accurate representation. With an updated conceptualisation of working memory based on Baddeley's (2000) work integrated in the model, Figure 5.3 presents a contemporary depiction of how memory is considered to operate. The model outlines memory processes. The different boxes suggest coordinated activities, but it is essential to remember that these activities, just like with consciousness, do not take place in one location in the brain (Miyake *et al.*, 2000).

First, all incoming information is processed in **sensory memory**. This is a network that holds on to sensory information for no longer than a second or so to enable unified further processing in the brain. It works in an autonomic way, so we have virtually no control over it.

Short-term memory or working memory

If we pay attention, the information will be transferred to **short-term memory (STM)** or **working memory**. Short-term memory involves an integration facility of limited capacity in which information can be retained and recalled for a period of several seconds to about a minute without being repeated. The capacity of STM was first researched by Miller (Miller, 1956) who suggested that, on average, humans can contain about seven different items, plus or minus two, at any one time in STM. If new information comes in, items entered earlier may be replaced. Such items are, for instance, sounds or visual images. You become aware of the size of STM when someone calls out a telephone number to you. It is usually after about seven to nine numbers that you realise that the last numbers are not retained or that the first numbers are replaced. By continuing to repeat the numbers, we may retain more.

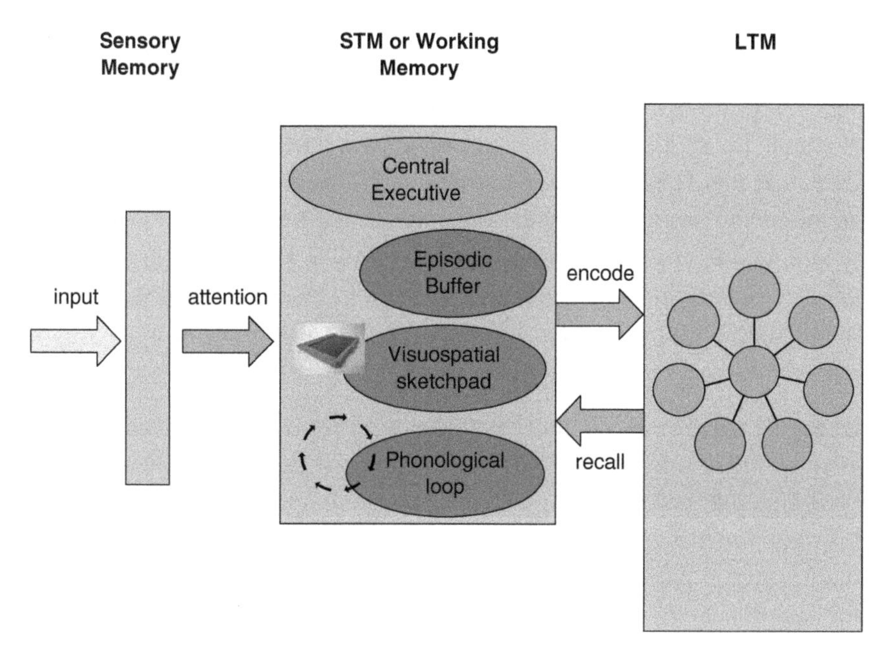

Figure 5.3: Integrated model of memory

Baddeley proposed the use of the term 'working memory' to emphasise that STM is also used in recalling existing memories. He suggested that working memory consists of a so-called 'phonological loop' for sounds and a 'visuospatial sketchpad' for visual and spatial information (Baddeley and Hitch, 1974). Furthermore, he proposed an active system that combines and channels attention and compares new information with what we already know. He refers to this as the 'central executive'. The principle of the central executive seems most closely related to what we consider consciousness or a 'thinking' process. More recently, Baddeley added an 'episodic buffer' to this model based on research that showed that people with amnesia for sounds and vision were still able to recall a storyline or sequence of events (Baddeley, 2000). The limited size of working memory is the main limitation to our thinking and consciousness. However, the active use of the four modules integrated in working memory will allow more efficient use of it.

Activity 5.2 — *Critical thinking*

How could you optimise your short term or working memory?

You are present at an intake session for a day centre for older adults. You don't have your notepad, but would like to remember details. Look up more detail on Baddeley's four working memory processes (on-line) and outline how to bring them under your control to make more effective use of them:

- central executive;
- phonological loop;
- visuospatial sketchpad;
- episodic buffer.

An outline answer is provided at the end of the chapter.

Long-term memory (LTM)

The consolidation process presented above is at the basis of **encoding** in long-term memory. Of course to reactivate, i.e. recall, information in long-term memory, it is essential that encoding has been done in a way that facilitates this. In general, effort put into connecting new information with existing knowledge, associating it with similar information, and using more than one medium to store the information, makes it more likely that we will be able to recall or recognise it when we want access to the information. Generating mind-maps helps provide a structure to information that can help both storage and recall. Within LTM the distinction is usually made between separate types of information which may or may not be stored as part of separate processes.

Explicit memory or declarative memory includes what we consciously know. Within explicit memory there are three sub systems. 'Episodic memory' is representing events, sequences and narratives (Tulving, 2002). Overlapping with this, 'autobiographical memory' includes what happened in your life. You may be able to remember events that happened earlier on the same day, but also what happened months or years ago. Many of these memories may not be recalled at will, but through association or prompting ('Do you remember when you performed your first CPR? That was when you were still a student'). Autobiographical memories give us a sense of continuity about our lives. The full consolidation of episodic memory is not present early in life. Hence, we don't have explicit recall of what happened when we were infants or toddlers. The third subsystem is 'semantic memory', which includes all else we know and understand.

Implicit memory contains what we are not consciously aware of. Within implicit memory distinction is often made between 'procedural memory', which includes the muscle and coordination memory for how to ride a bike and other procedures. It also contains 'emotional memory', which is activated to store memories of strong emotions, often in conjunction with episodic memory. Perhaps these distinctions should not be taken as meaning that there are entirely separate processes or neural modules involved. The reality is that, in many cases, these different types of long-term memory may be intertwined. As more associations are available, recall will be more effective, although we should never expect perfect reproduction of what was experienced or learned (see True or False video in Useful websites).

Activity 5.3 *Reflection*

Memories of your first placement.

Can you identify an example of each type of long term memory (LTM) related to your first placement?

Type of long term memory		Your example
Explicit or declarative	*Episodic memory*	
	Autobiographical memory	
	Semantic memory	
Implicit memory	*Procedural memory*	
	Emotional memory	

Forgetting

First and foremost, we forget as a result of neural wear and tear. This process can become problematic later on in life. Often the issue is not that the information has disappeared, but that the pathways to find it may have become less accessible. Secondly, our neural connections in the brain are subject to a process of neural 'pruning' (see Chapter 4). This is a normal process that allows us to make quicker decisions and act faster, because we process less irrelevant information. Generally, information that has been encoded in several modalities (visual, auditory, verbal, and kinaesthetic, etc.) will remain more accessible. Also, information that has been retrieved often and therefore has been stored repeatedly will be more easily accessible. Furthermore, specific memories can be repressed because thinking of them is unpleasant or traumatic.

When you are **studying** you may experience that there may be interference during the encoding process. New learning may interfere with the retention of material that has been addressed just before (retroactive forgetting). Or the opposite may take place, with what you've just tried to memorise interfering with retaining new material (proactive forgetting). These processes can make an evening among the books rather disappointing and stressful. They also affect how well you remember a lecture. Typically your STM may get flooded and your encoding may be unable to keep up when a lecturer operates at high speed and does not leave space to reflect and make associations to effectively encode material in LTM. In a sense it is probably correct to say that a lot of what we think gets forgotten, perhaps never gets encoded well enough. We would argue that effective use of your memory is most crucial at the moment of learning. Without paying proper attention, a specific aspect may not get encoded in LTM. For instance, when you meet a new patient, you shake hands and names are exchanged, but you realise that, moments later, you have forgotten the name. The same thing happens at parties. We don't like it because we consider it evidence of lack of interest. Here is an exercise to come to a better understanding of why this happens and what you can do about it (see Activity 5.4).

Activity 5.4 *Evidence-based practice and research*

Remembering names (this works best with a group of 15-25 students).

Instructions:

1. Each student adopts a new first name (don't tell anyone yet, write it down on a piece of paper and put in your pocket).
2. All students get up and walk around the classroom, shake everybody's hand while saying their NEW first name to each other, until done.
3. Test: let everybody stand up in order, number them, and let students write down their NEW name.
4. Students reveal their NEW names and check who had the most correct answers.

Discuss afterwards:

- What did the most effective students do to remember the names?
- Reflect on what the experts say (see Useful websites).

Memory and memory loss in your patients

As we've seen in Chapter 4, the precision of our memory or memory 'fidelity' declines with age (Benjamin, 2010). It is a general and gradual decline. Most people find ways of compensating by paying more attention and putting more effort into encoding. Overall, it seems inevitable, but caregivers can assist older patients by providing contextual information, cues and reminders (May *et al.*, 2005). This kind of support can also reduce the impact of dementia in your patients. In most cases, when consciousness is affected so is memory. When your patients have been in an accident it is not uncommon for them to have limited memory of events, particularly if they lost consciousness (Mayou *et al.*, 2000, Murray *et al.*, 2002). Often they don't remember the accident or part of what happened. Similarly, victims of violent crime will often not remember features of their assailant, in particular if a weapon was used (Steblay, 1992). Research on soldiers in combat has also provided solid evidence on memory loss as part of a traumatic reaction (Van der Kolk and McFarlane, 2012). Our natural tendency is to try and fill in the blanks. This process is, as you will understand from the above, fraught with difficulties. Research on alcohol-induced memory loss has shown that it is quite likely that events are not reconstructed accurately (Nash and Takarangi, 2011).

On a different note, there are of course things we don't want to remember, such as an operation. While rare, there are some documented cases in which a comprehensive anaesthetic had not entirely inhibited memory formation at an implicit level (Schwender *et al.*, 1994). This can be confusing, if not traumatic, for the patient.

False memories

When our fate and that of other people relies on our memory, it is of particular importance that it can be trusted. Unfortunately, there is a lot of evidence that our memories are quite prone to include false elements or essential mistakes (Schacter, 1999; Loftus, 2005; Schacter and Addis, 2007). Sometimes memories have been shown to be entirely wrong. In such cases, the person was often convinced that their memories accurately presented what had happened. As a result of this, people have gone to prison falsely accused (Loftus, 1996). Families have been torn apart by accounts of child abuse that emerged from overly zealous and suggestive interview techniques used by child psychologists (Loftus and Ketcham, 1996; London *et al.*, 2005) or suggestive reflective strategies in psychotherapists (Clancy *et al.*, 2000). We have arguments with our colleagues about what happened and who did what when mistakes are made in hospital. The essence is that memories are malleable, sometimes biased towards self-protection, affected by stress, anger, fear, love or other emotions and, once we've told someone about it, the way we've told it will affect our memory of the initial event.

Concept summary: Ways of improving memory

You can improve your memory in the following ways:

1. Paying conscious attention and avoiding distraction helps your STM.
2. Allowing the encoding process in LTM to catch up every now and again by taking a small break in which you do nothing other than reflect.

3. By connecting the information to be learned to related knowledge and by using multiple ways of encoding in LTM you will be more likely to reproduce the material. The visual, auditory and language (written and spoken) aspect each make use of additional channels that add to the representation of the material in the brain.
4. Do something actively such as using mnemonics, making notes, repeating it, or executing any movements (kinaesthetic processing) related to the learning. You will be much more effective in retaining it.
5. Creativity and effort used at the learning stage (encoding) will pay itself back at the exam (recall) stage.
6. Use mind-mapping to create a meaningful organisation of associations in the material you want to remember. You will see that this will function as 'pull down menus' during recall.
7. Prepare reminders for recall during learning (when you see this > remember that).
8. Each time you review, recall or use what you memorised you reactivate the material and encode an additional version. It is like you are telling your brain, 'Don't forget this yet, we are using this!'

Optimising your memory

It is essential to see that the strength of your memory of an event is based on conscious attention, active effort and creativity put into encoding, the extent of the review of the event afterwards, elapsed time between recall and previous recall, and avoiding interference with other information. If you are interested in learning more about techniques to improve your memory it will be worthwhile to look up the work of Tony Buzan (Buzan, 2006) or investigate what you can pick up from Neuro-linguistic Programming (NLP) (Adler, 2002). There are also many specific materials and mnemonics (memory aids) available for nurses (see Useful websites). To finish the chapter we have one more activity for you, to help you imagine and hopefully put to the test what you've learned about the effective use of your memory.

Activity 5.5 — *Critical thinking*

Describe how you will optimise memory in the following examples.

Task	Attention and focus	Effective encoding in multiple modalities	Reviewing
Example: You are instructed in a new hand-over approach on the computer.	*Make sure you sit straight in front of the screen; remove all distractions; rehearse material as you are learning it.*	*Do the navigation yourself (kinaesthetic); insist on verbal and visual instruction; repeat all moves and make notes of key instructions.*	*The moment you have a chance, practise the use of the new system several times.*

continued . . .

continued . . .

Task	Attention and focus	Effective encoding in multiple modalities	Reviewing
1. You are new on a ward and want to remember the names of your colleagues.			
2. A new defibrillator has arrived and you receive instructions in its use.			
3. You are studying this chapter in preparation for a test or exam.			

An outline answer is provided at the end of the chapter.

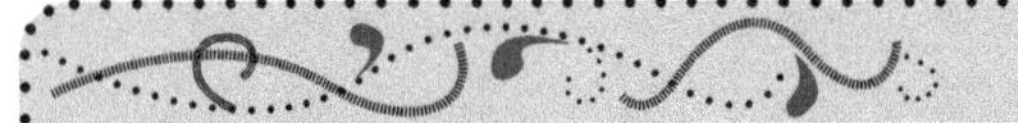

Chapter summary

- Consciousness requires concentration and effort and is essential for planning, decision making, problem solving and reflection.
- We've identified four levels of consciousness according to the degree of intentional activity involved.
- It is important to be aware of sleep patterns (REM sleep and deep sleep), because it will allow you to have a better understanding of your patients' and your own ability to cope with daily pressure.
- Both consciousness and memory have clear constraints that constitute the main bottleneck for intelligent processing of information. We can only focus on a limited number of things at one time.
- Memory can be unreliable and is prone to being affected by inattention, false memories, tiredness, and forgetting.
- There are many ways in which you can make more effective use of your memory. It is worth investigating this (see Further reading and Useful websites).

Activities: brief outline answers

Scenario: Consciousness and distraction (see page 78)

Sue may need to promise herself to call her mother during her next break. If this does not help, she could make a quick call to apologise and take the urgency away. This way she may be able to concentrate again.

Scenario: Consciousness and experience (see page 78)

When tasks are not automated they cannot be executed while having a conversation. You would need to stop the blood pressure procedure as you converse and resume the task when the conversation comes to a pause. It is okay to explain this to patients. They will understand.

Activity 5.1 (see page 80)

Multi-tasking – most likely level 3 with automated activities competing for attention; *full anaesthetic* – not conscious; *routine activities* – level 3 or 4; *profound intellectual disability* – unknown; *coma* – not conscious but not always certain of this; *locked in syndrome* – consciousness possible at all levels; *meditating or* praying – alternate consciousness, not one of the four levels; *mind altering drugs* – alternate consciousness, not one of the four levels; *before and after birth* – perhaps level 1 or 2, but not really known; *severe dementia* – all four levels but probably with many flaws.

Case study: Overcoming helplessness (see page 81)

The nurse needs to get Mary to start doing things for herself again. She may challenge Mary with activities that require high levels of consciousness. A step-by-step approach may be essential to ensure this approach succeeds.

Scenario: How have you slept? (see page 83)

Maintaining and restoring regularity in sleeping patterns (sleeping hygiene) is essential to avoid insomnia or non-restorative sleep at night. Reducing noise in the clinical environment is important, including ensuring that nurses, if chatting, keep noise to a minimum. If possible, physical and mental activity during the day may improve sleep at night. Review all medication that leads to sleep deprivation.

Activity 5.2 (see page 85)

Central executive – reflect on how information you receive relates to your knowledge and experiences; *phonological loop* – can be actively used by repeating important names and terms; *visuospatial sketchpad* – take note of what those present look like, what they are wearing, where they are in the room, etc.; *episodic buffer* – keep track of sequence of events and try to remember stories.

Activity 5.3 (see page 86)

Examples should be personal and help you identify the different types of LTM.

Activity 5.4 (see page 87)

In general students who put creative effort into memorising the names will have been more effective.

Activity 5.5 (see page 89)

Task 1: force yourself to pay attention to the names. Repeat them, see them written down, say the names and repeat the names whenever you can. Write them down and review several times. *Task 2*: sit close and pay active attention, ask questions, volunteer to try things out, if unsure of something insist on being allowed to try again, make notes and review afterwards, ensure that confusion with previous equipment is resolved. *Task 3*: pay attention, study in periods of about 25 minutes and 2–3 minute breaks, do all assignments to make the material come alive; copy Figure 5.1, 5.2, Table 5.2, and review actively.

Further reading

Dennett, Daniel (1993) *Consciousness explained.* London, UK: Penguin.

This is still one of the most readable and insightful books on consciousness ever written.

Buzan, Tony (2010) *Use your head: how to unleash the power of your mind.* London: BBC Pearson.

Most books by Buzan give hope to all of us who spend too much time chasing after memories and possessions we consider lost.

Loftus, E. F. (2005) Planting misinformation in the human mind: a 30-year investigation of the malleability of memory. *Learning & Memory*, 12(4): 361–366.

This is a useful introduction to how unreliable our memory may be. Also look for Elizabeth Loftus' lectures on-line.

Useful websites

http://www.kidsmathgamesonline.com/memory/simon.html

The Simon Says game provides an excellent opportunity to explore how your short term or working memory operates for you.

http://www.memorise.org/memory-training/secrets-remembering-names-00925.html

This website provides expert advice on how you can improve your memory.

http://www.youtube.com/watch?v=4lisNg91_M0

True or False: this Scientific American Frontiers video shows research by noted memory researcher Dan Schacter (and the actor Alan Alda) on false memories, and provides an excellent explanation of how memory works.

https://www.pinterest.com/pin/23362491794560033/

This website provides apps and memory supports for nurses.

Chapter 6
Thinking, motivation, feeling, action

Chapter aims

After reading this chapter you will be able to:

- explain the core processes involved in thinking (cognition), motivation and feeling (emotion);
- discuss the implications and provide examples of how we think in both highly sophisticated, and simplistic and stereotypical ways;
- understand how we solve problems and what our strengths and limitations are in addressing problems in health care;
- understand and apply the mechanisms of motivation and emotion to nurses and patients;
- describe how thoughts, motivation and feelings are interacting in nursing care.

Nurses need to be highly motivated, think on their feet and deal effectively with patients' emotions and their own. This chapter looks at the processes and mechanisms involved. We address cognition, with specific focus on the distinction between thinking in complex and simplistic ways. As regards motivation, the focus is on what drives us and how needs are prioritised. Emotions are covered by addressing a variety of theoretical perspectives. Eventually the interaction between thinking, emotions, motivation and behaviour is addressed, including what happens when we experience inconsistency.

Thinking (cognition)

When we use the term 'thinking' we normally mean a conscious process. However, as we know from the previous chapter, much of our processing in the brain is not conscious. To ensure that we include this in our understanding, psychologists use the term 'cognition' as an overarching term for all thinking and knowing, regardless of whether we are aware of it or not. It includes understanding, reasoning, appraisal, problem solving, reflecting, remembering, as well as complex, simplistic and automatic information processing. We do some of our thinking in words and sentences, but we also think in associations, numbers, movement, images, sounds and other sensations. Furthermore, we think in concepts, principles and beliefs. Impressive, isn't it? No wonder we consider ourselves 'Rational Wonders'. Unfortunately, there is considerable evidence that we often don't operate in this way and instead use shortcuts, stereotypes, imprecise, sloppy and simplistic approaches in our thinking. Fiske and Taylor introduced the term 'Cognitive

Miser' (Fiske, 2004; Fiske and Taylor, 1991) for this type of thinking. To appreciate the full spectrum of our cognitive abilities we need to be cognisant of both of these ways of thinking. The scenario below provides a comparison.

Scenario: Rational Wonder and Cognitive Miser in nursing

The Rational Wonder in nursing

Imagine you are working in intensive care. You are responsible for patients with multiple invasive technologies, who require continuous monitoring and have complex care needs. You need to be responsive to progress and deterioration in conditions, monitor equipment, and intervene when appropriate. To do this effectively you need to think accurately and clearly, prioritise, make rational and balanced decisions, and expertly combine a variety of sources of information and knowledge. It includes multi-tasking, and you need to be fully awake and have the ambition to perform as well as possible. If you recognise yourself in this description you know what it is like to operate as a Rational Wonder. When you are in this 'mode' of operation you have access to the best of your mental abilities. You feel tired after a day like this, but it is also rewarding to think that you are performing as well as you can.

The Cognitive Miser in nursing

Consider yourself working in the same environment on a different day. There has been a problem with the staffing and you are now finding yourself responsible for the care of several more patients than the day before. To compound the situation a few patients require more attention than you can give. You find yourself stressed and overwhelmed. You are making instant decisions on whose care needs to be prioritised but, in the next moment, you have to overturn these decisions. Everything has to be done fast. It is not unlikely that in these circumstances you take shortcuts in your assessment, make intuitive decisions about the seriousness of someone's condition, and allow yourself very little time to think things through. When you are in this mode of operation, you are much more likely to make mistakes. At the end of your shift, you realise that the Cognitive Miser in you may have taken over a few times. How would you feel?

An outline response is provided at the end of the chapter.

Comparing Rational Wonder with Cognitive Miser (see Table 6.1)

We have both of these modes of operation within us. Whether we'll be operating in one or the other depends on the pressure of circumstances, but also on your own energy and motivation. The Rational Wonder way requires more mental effort and a higher complexity and sophistication in our thinking. We may be under pressure but, when we are alert, well rested and able for the job, we will activate this mode of operation. Typically, when we are overexcited, overloaded, tired, worried, low in motivation or under too much time pressure, the Cognitive Miser in us may

Table 6.1: Rational Wonder *vs* Cognitive Miser modes

Rational Wonder	Cognitive Miser
Complex thinking, using your intelligence	Simplistic thinking
Thinking through a problem	Trial-and-error problem solving
High mental effort	Low mental effort
Precise assessments and decision making	Imprecise intuitions in decision making
Original and creative solutions	Standard solutions
Nuanced and balanced thinking	Stereotypical thinking
Resisting bias and prejudice	Acting on biased and prejudiced thinking
Well-paced activity including reflection	Hurried activity without reflection

prevail. In an environment where people's lives depend on accuracy it is essential to be aware of when thinking shifts into Cognitive Miser mode. You can check your understanding of the distinction between Rational Wonder and Cognitive Miser thinking in Table 6.1 and Activity 6.1.

Several researchers have proposed similarly focused cognitive dichotomies. Petty and Cacioppo's (1986) distinction between central and peripheral processing has perhaps been the most influential. They defined 'central processing' as thinking in depth based on a detailed analysis of several aspects of the information received. In contrast 'peripheral processing' was observed as based on the attractiveness and emotional impact of information. An almost identical distinction – between 'deep' and 'surface' processing – has emerged in education (Dinsmore and Alexander, 2012). Likewise, Nobel Prize winner Daniel Kahneman proposed the conceptualisation of 'fast and slow thinking', with slow and deep analysis on the one hand, and fast intuition and gut feelings on the other hand (Kahneman, 2011). While Kahneman argues that there is a time and place for both approaches to thinking, we would be against advocating the use of the fast system of thinking in health care.

Activity 6.1 *Critical thinking*

Indicate whether the examples fit in mostly with the Rational Wonder or Cognitive Miser way of thinking	Rational Wonder	Cognitive Miser
1. You change your ideas on how to treat patients with leg ulcers on the basis of a story a fellow nurse told you.		
2. You don't trust the computations for the dosage of the new medication for a patient and decide to compute it yourself.		

continued . . .

continued . . .

Indicate whether the examples fit in mostly with the Rational Wonder or Cognitive Miser way of thinking	Rational Wonder	Cognitive Miser
3. You need to fit a new endotracheal tube for a patient, but you don't know the diameter. You decide to try one that looks more or less the right size.		
4. A patient asks you what the evidence is for the use of homeopathy for muscle pain. You don't really know, but you advise against it.		
5. A young woman in your care shows signs of a heart attack. You think this is unlikely but, nonetheless, you ensure that this is looked into immediately by the resident cardiologist.		
6. Some handover information seems to be missing for a patient. You decide the patient looks fine and do not follow up on it.		
7. You fear an outbreak of a dangerous and contagious virus. You decide to isolate the wards, yourself and colleagues. Your next step is that you ensure all who've recently visited are contacted and advised to immediately see a doctor.		
8. You receive temperature information in Fahrenheit when you normally receive this information in Celsius. You decide to look up the exact conversion algorithm.		
9. You hear about exciting new evidence for the treatment of eating disorders. Since you work with adolescents with anorexia you decide to look it up in the research databases to which you have access. When you can't find it, you ask the hospital librarian to look it up for you.		
10. A patient from another country tries to let you know that there is something not right with the meal he received. You assume it is because the food is unusual to him.		

An outline answer is provided at the end of the chapter.

Thinking effort

High or low thinking effort is at the core of each of the distinctions discussed in the above. Thinking effort is experienced when our working memory is stretched (Backs and Seljos, 1994), as we've seen in the previous chapter. It is an adaptive warning signal. We tend to be acutely aware of it (Mulder, 1986) and are quite prepared to reduce energy expenditure, especially in the face of a lost cause. We are sure you've tried to solve a crossword, Sudoku, or another puzzle and hit a mental wall. At this point you had to decide whether you were prepared to increase your efforts or give up. In the case of a crossword there is not much at stake, so throwing in the towel is OK. However, if you have a pressing and highly complex nursing problem you are not in a position to give up. Also, while you might be tempted to save energy and make a quick but not well-considered decision (Cognitive Miser) it is essential that you use the 'effort' signal to warn yourself to resist and maintain the Rational Wonder approach.

Calm thinking and problem solving

Remaining calm helps significantly in maintaining rationality. You will likely see very good examples of this in health care. Doctors, nurses, midwives, and other healthcare professionals are often incredibly adept at remaining calm under pressure. Maintaining a calm composure counteracts over-arousal (as we've seen in the 'Running around' scenario in Chapter 3, see page 40) and this ultimately benefits performance (Yerkes and Dodson, 1908) including rational thinking. Intense emotions and over-arousal tend to trigger typical thinking obstacles such as:

a. **Functional fixedness**: we get overly fixated on the regular way in which something is done or used and overlook alternative possibilities.
b. **Mental set (rigidity)**: we fail to adapt our method of reasoning when we are not successful.
c. **Unnecessary constraints**: we imagine limitations that are not there.
d. **Overemphasis on irrelevant information**: we fail to see the kernel of the problem as a result of being unable to identify what is essential and what is not.

(Weiten, 2010).

This is not to say that all problem solving has to be devoid of emotion. Motivation, and the energy that comes with this, is more important than you might think. In fact, there are problems we seem to be better at resolving because they upset us. There is evidence that unfairness or cheating tend to activate superior problem-solving abilities (Cosmides and Tooby, 1992; Cosmides, 1989).

Creative thinking

Effective problem solving also tends to benefit from creative thinking. Contemporary lingo has given us the phrase 'thinking outside of the box'! Creative problem solving is the ability to see original and new solutions or to rephrase a problem in a new way to enable its solution. Creative reasoning is often considered the epitome of sophistication in thinking (Coon and Mitterer, 2012). In health care, creative problem solving is associated with better governance and improved patient care (Motamedi, 2012; DiCenso *et al.*, 2010; Plsek and Wilson, 2001). Creativity is often essential to address problems that have been highly resistant to being resolved. Interestingly, Zedelius and Schooler (Zedelius and Schooler, 2015) questioned whether a focused (mindful) or a wandering mind (mindless) would be most conducive to creativity. Their experiments showed that creativity involving analysis benefits from the focus of mindfulness, while creativity involving insight benefits from a wandering mind. This makes sense. Some of the greatest scientists and artists have admitted that major ideas or theories simply came to them as 'aha' moments, and even in dreams.

Scenarios: Creative problem solving

Can you identify the core ideas in how problems are solved in these two scenarios?

Frequent medication errors were a matter of grave concern in the small hospital in which Siobhan worked. During a brainstorm in the multi-disciplinary team, she suggested that mistakes could be prevented if medications starting with the same letter were not placed next to one another. The hospital pharmacy department decided that although drugs had always been shelved alphabetically, they could be reorganised by drug type. Following this, errors were greatly reduced.	*Harry is a children's nurse who had to separate two boys who were fighting over toys, a digger and a truck. Another nurse had given the digger to one boy and the truck to the other, but they felt that they could not play with them separately. Harry invented a story in which digger and truck came from two different planets and had to learn to help each other. This taught the boys to play together and they had more fun this way.*

An outline response is provided at the end of the chapter.

The power of positive thinking

Being optimistic tends to have a powerful positive impact on our functioning (Carver *et al.*, 2010; Scheier and Carver, 1993). Cognitive processes play an important role in this, as research in Positive Psychology suggests (Seligman, 2011). Positive expectations accompanied by imagining successful outcomes may even work as self-fulfilling prophecies. This is of importance to nurses and patients alike. If you think 'I can do it' you set in motion a mechanism whereby positive thinking, positive feelings, and success-focused action tendencies interact in favourable ways (see Figure 6.1).

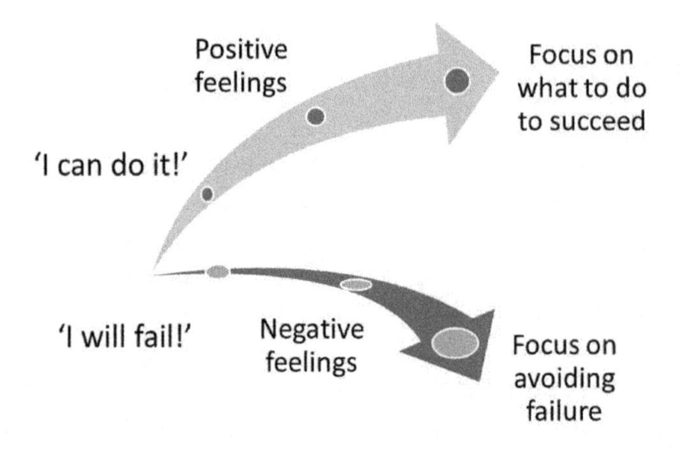

Figure 6.1: The power of positive thinking

In contrast, thinking 'I will fail' will generate negative feelings and a failure-oriented action focus which is more stressful and quite likely detrimental to performance levels. Of particular concern is that we may be conditioned to think in negative ways without being aware of it. To change this requires effort and practice. It may necessitate consciously adopting a more optimistic perspective and reminding oneself often to think positive thoughts. Obvious benefits for our mood will reinforce the motivation to make this our dominant mode of operation.

Critical thinking or reflection in nurses

While positivity is a powerful asset, nurses also need to think and reflect critically on their work (Bandman and Bandman, 1988; Jasper, 2013) in order to maintain high standards. Without this, optimism and positivity would become a liability. It is most likely that reflection is taught as part of nursing education. Exactly how is still a matter of dispute. In our view critical reflection in nursing needs to include a preparedness to find fault with one's own clinical practice by comparing it with nursing values, standards and regulations. Also, if we fail to meet expected levels, action needs to be taken to do something about this. It is important to recognise that a thought process ('level of care is not up to scratch') leads to an emotion (being upset) that, in turn, motivates behavioural change (practice improvement) (de Vries and Timmins, 2016). We will come back to this later in the chapter when we discuss how inconsistency motivates us. Let us discuss motivation in more detail now.

Motivation

Considering how demanding nursing is, it is important that you are highly motivated. With a strong motivation you are more likely to be able to cope with the responsibility, the pressure and the long hours. The type of motivation also matters. Psychologists tend to distinguish between **extrinsic motivation**, when you do something motivated by outside rewards, and **intrinsic motivation**, when you do something motivated by the satisfaction you derive from the activity itself. The literature suggests that the latter is more effective at keeping people going in long term and potentially stressful endeavours such as a nursing job (Janssen *et al.*, 1999). Traditionally, when religious orders ran hospitals, nursing was seen as a vocation, which is the ultimate intrinsic motivation. Even today there are voices that suggest that the nursing profession is a calling (Heyes, 2005). It may be interesting to consider your own motivation.

Scenario: Nurse motivation

You talk with fellow students about what motivates you as a nurse. Bukola says she considers herself mostly motivated by helping and supporting others, and the thought that she will have an opportunity to make a difference in other people's lives. She says she suspects she is well suited for a nursing job because she is really interested in health and medical science, and the idea of working for a hospital or other health-care organisation appeals to her. In contrast, Rita says that she is simply looking for a way

continued . . .

continued . . .

of earning a decent living and being respected by others for studying something that is most likely to ensure she will have a job. Discuss their motivations (and your own) in relation to the issue of intrinsic and extrinsic motivation.

An outline response is provided at the end of the chapter.

In addition, you may wonder what motivates the people in your care, their family members and perhaps, more broadly, what drives people in general. Let's have a look at what psychological theory says about this.

Drive reduction theory

In its most essential form, motivation is the energy or 'the influences that account for the initiation, direction, intensity, and persistence of behaviour' (Bernstein *et al.*, 2012, p. 407). What motivates people's activities can be complex but also based on very basic needs. This is how it works according to 'drive reduction theory' (see Figure 6.2).

Our system has many needs that must be fulfilled to be in balance. We are alerted when a need is not fulfilled (Hull, 1943). This is often felt as unpleasant. Hull called it a 'drive', which motivates behaviour aimed at reducing the drive. So if we lack nutrition or fluids we experience the drive of hunger or thirst, which motivates eating or drinking until we've had enough. At that point a feedback mechanism kicks in that reduces the drive. With the reduction of the urge we would normally stop eating or drinking. Thus homeostasis for nutrients or fluids in the body is re-established. While the homeostasis principle may not be applicable beyond hunger and thirst,

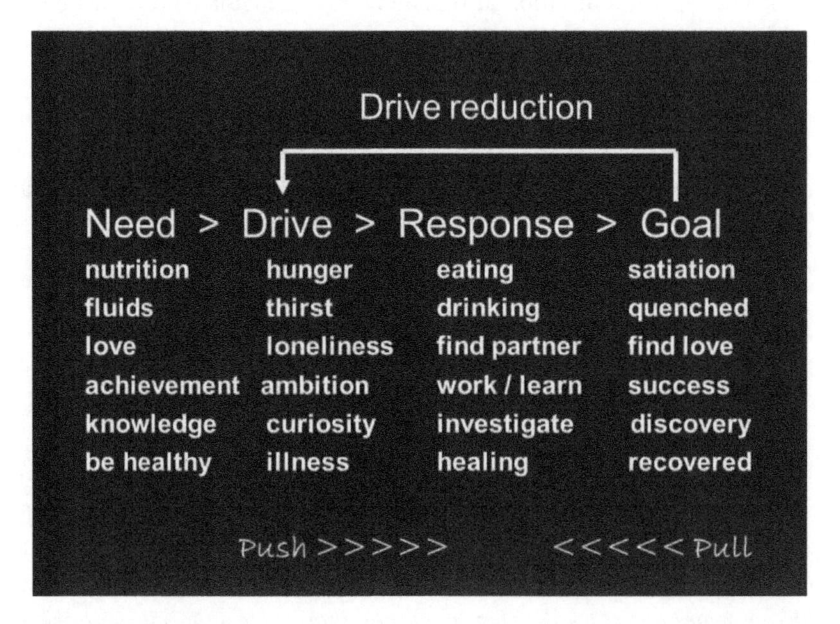

Figure 6.2: Drive reduction theory

we can easily see the relevance of drive reduction for more complex needs such as love and achievement. If we really want we could even fit in the need to be healthy, with illness as a drive, seeking healing as a response, and recovery as a goal.

The drive reduction mechanism is essential for the model but also a limiting element. For instance, ask yourself how often being successful at something leads to a reduction of your ambition. It may, but your success may also reinforce your ambition. Another question mark about the model is that it emphasises that we are 'pushed' by drives though, perhaps just as often, we are 'pulled' into activities by the imminence of a goal. You may not think of eating until there is food in front of you. You may not feel ambitious until there is an opportunity to achieve a success. You may not feel lonely until you suddenly run into someone you consider the love of your life (in which case you had better do something). In short, motivation is more complex than the principle of drive reduction suggests.

Hierarchy of Needs

A particularly interesting issue is that we tend to experience many drives at the same time. How do we prioritise attending to them? *Maslow's Hierarchy of Needs* (Maslow, 1943) suggests that we are inclined to attend to physiological needs before more higher order needs (see Figure 6.3). In the model, safety is a second priority after physical needs, followed by love and belonging, esteem and self-esteem, and the principle of 'self-actualisation', generally considered the motivation to give meaning to life. If you take the model literally you would perhaps conclude that unless physiological and safety needs are addressed we cannot attend to 'belonging' and the higher needs. As a thinking exercise, try to establish exceptions to this idea. In some depictions of the pyramid 'sex' is included among the physiological needs, but should that mean that you cannot focus on more higher order needs if you have not had sex?

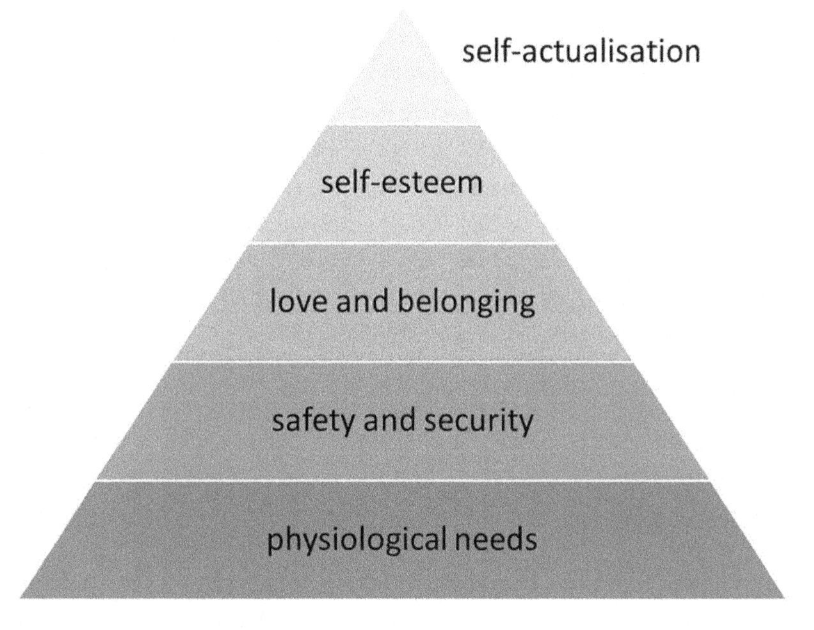

Figure 6.3: Maslow's Hierarchy of Needs

Another limitation of the model is that it does not include 'having children'. Where could that fit in, if you wanted to include it? Furthermore, Maslow himself noted the omission of the need for 'knowledge' and added it later (Maslow *et al.*, 1970). Several other authors have also tinkered with the model as you will see if you look up depictions online. A final, not so minor, problem is that empirical verification of such a complex model is almost impossible. Funnily enough, none of this seems to deter nursing educators from considering Maslow's model as particularly relevant to nurses.

Perhaps the main reason we are still addressing Maslow's model is that, with the principle of **self-actualisation**, it has highlighted the idea that people are motivated to use their talents and strive towards becoming who or what they want to be. Like with the model as a whole, the term has been reinterpreted and expanded, perhaps because it makes sense to well-fed people with high expectations and many choices in an ambitious society. Contemporary authors usually emphasise that self-actualisation is a process rather than a goal that you can reach. Nurses (Hsu, 2015) and patients (Kehyayan *et al.*, 2015) who engaged in self-actualisation were likely to experience a higher quality of life. The model can be used by nurses to consider their own motivation. For instance, an analysis of how much time and effort is devoted to each level of need on an average day can be very revealing. The model can also help establish the extent to which the needs of patients and families are satisfied (Kosco and Warren, 2000). Furthermore, patients' motivation to actively contribute to getting well may be analysed with the model. In some cases, when patients do not seem to want to leave the hospital, one may wonder whether going home would be jeopardising their physiological needs, safety or self-esteem.

Scenario: New purpose-built psychiatric unit

A new purpose-built psychiatric unit has an open plan style, using a 'hub and spoke' model with an open nurses' station in the centre. Architecture and design were state of the art and aimed at creating a light and friendly environment. Nurses were encouraged to engage more with clients and the use of seclusion and locking clients' bedroom doors (other than at night) was discouraged. The environment was working out reasonably well, although lack of tea- and lunch-making facilities in the hub (for safety reasons) was considered a drawback. A quality inspection was critical when they found that nurses were spending a lot of their time in a kitchen away from the scene instead of at the hub of the unit. A subsequent investigation revealed that the new open-plan unit had left staff feeling vulnerable, unsafe and in need of more privacy. Management used Maslow's Hierarchy of Needs in their considerations regarding what to do. Can you imagine their discussions?

An outline response is provided at the end of the chapter.

Complex motivation

Drive Reduction Theory and the Hierarchy of Needs together provide a meaningful way of understanding motivation. However, reality is complex and requires us to think and strategise to wisely devote energy to satisfy the myriad of needs we have. The more intricate this becomes the more cognitive resources we use to navigate effectively in life. To complicate things further, activities may have multiple motivations and different drives may motivate contrary actions. Often motivational conflict seems inevitable and can make life hard for us. At the same time, it is important to emphasise – and let's move on to this now – that we do not only 'think' but also 'feel' our way through life and guide our activities with emotions as much as cognitions. Similar to drives, emotions can have a motivating function. When we feel joy this may motivate us to laugh and smile at others. When we feel fear it may motivate us to hide away. Let's take a closer look.

Emotions

Generally, when we talk about feelings, we discriminate between emotions and moods. Emotions are generally seen as more directly triggered by events and fluctuate frequently and rapidly, while moods tend to linger and persist over time. Emotions are composed of a subjective qualitative experience (positive or negative), accompanying physiological arousal (high or low), expressions (to communicate the emotion), accompanying thought patterns, and an action tendency or behavioural response (Bernstein *et al.*, 2012). So, if your emotion is joy, the experience is probably accompanied by high sympathetic arousal experienced as excitement; this may be expressed in smiling and lead to dancing around the table or other behavioural expressions. If your emotion is sadness, you are probably experiencing low sympathetic arousal, you may express it with a sad face or crying, and you may withdraw from company.

Basic or primary emotions

Many psychologists discriminate between emotions of the **excited** kind, such as joy, surprise, fear, anger, and emotions of the **inhibited** kind such as sadness and acceptance (Frijda, 1986). The way in which individuals feel and express emotions varies, and so is the extent to which we control or suppress them. This creates the impression that people have highly individualised emotions. Nonetheless, today many theorists subscribe to the idea that, in essence, our emotional 'palette' is limited to five to ten **primary emotions**, which are similarly experienced all over the world (Plutchik, 1980; Izard, 1992; Tooby and Cosmides, 1990; Ekman, 1992) (see Figure 6.4). Plutchik (1980) highlights eight primary emotions (sadness, disgust, anger, anticipation, joy, trust, fear, surprise), while Ekman (1992) suggests six (sadness, fear, disgust, surprise, anger, joy).

Basic emotions are seen to have evolved as adaptations in our efforts to survive and reproduce (Tooby and Cosmides, 2008). We should not be surprised that we are equipped with the propensity to experience strong fear because it helps us to avoid danger and thus aids our survival. Similarly, we are highly motivated to seek the pleasurable experience of joy and ecstasy, such as in sex, which promotes reproduction and thus the survival of our genes. An emotion organises our physiological and mental functioning and prioritises our activities. This even includes a mechanism whereby our facial expression is fed back to the brain and confirms and strengthens the emotion that is expressed (McIntosh, 1996). This implies that while we tend to think that we smile because we feel good, the opposite is also true. A good reason to remember to smile!

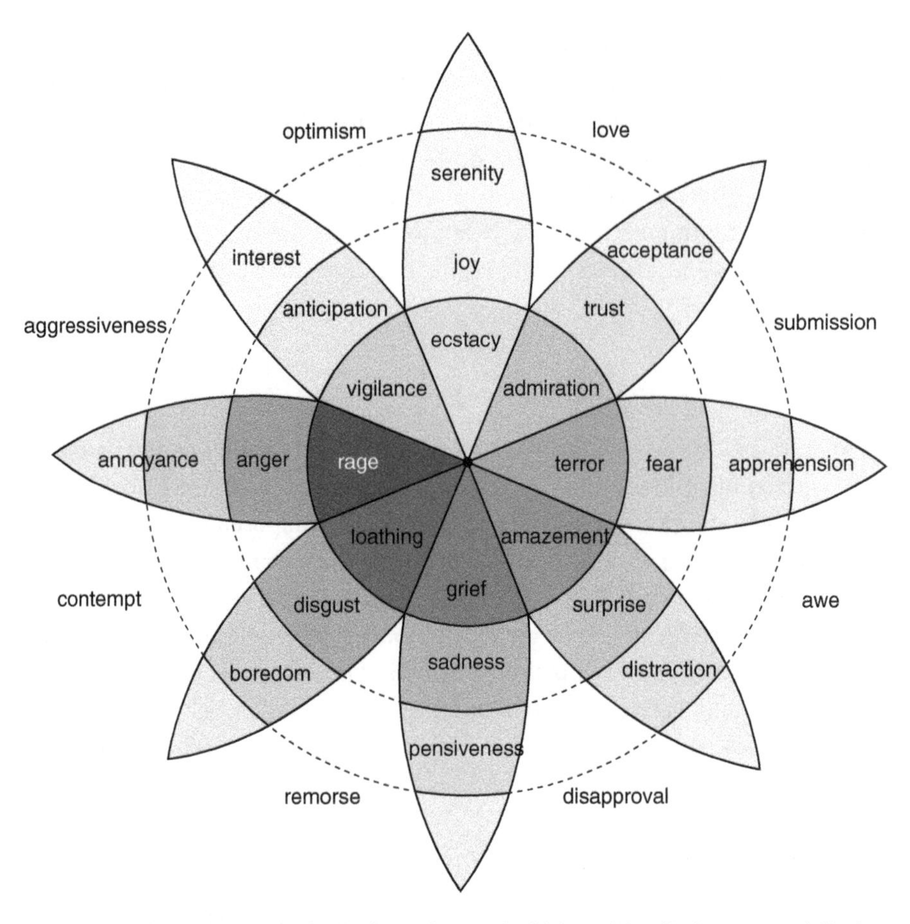

The eight emotions in the centre are the basic dimensions at the highest intensity (e.g. ecstasy). To the outside of the model the intensity fades to lesser degrees of the same emotional dimension (e.g. ecstasy, joy, serenity).

Figure 6.4: Primary Emotions (Plutchik, 1980)

Activity 6.2 ***Reflection***

Discuss Plutchik's eight basic emotions in Figure 6.4 (sadness, disgust, anger, anticipation, joy, trust, fear, surprise). Identify when you've experienced these emotions at different levels of intensity. Make notes of what you did to control your emotions and when you found it difficult. This should help you develop Emotional Intelligence (EQ) i.e. effective awareness, handling and expression of emotions and interpersonal relationships (Goleman, 1995).

An outline response is provided at the end of the chapter.

Emotions as communication

Emotions are not just about experience and expression. They are also a form of communication. If a patient expresses fear before an operation, it is important that a nurse recognises this from the facial and bodily expression, rather than having to wait for the patient to say 'Nurse, I am scared'. This way, the nurse can do something to reduce the fear at an earlier stage. In a way, the

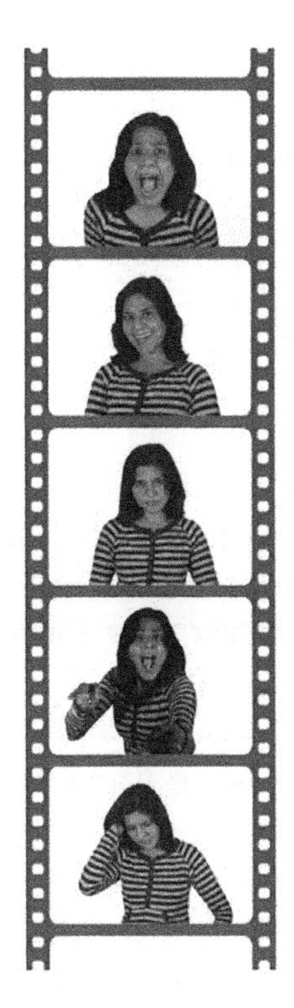

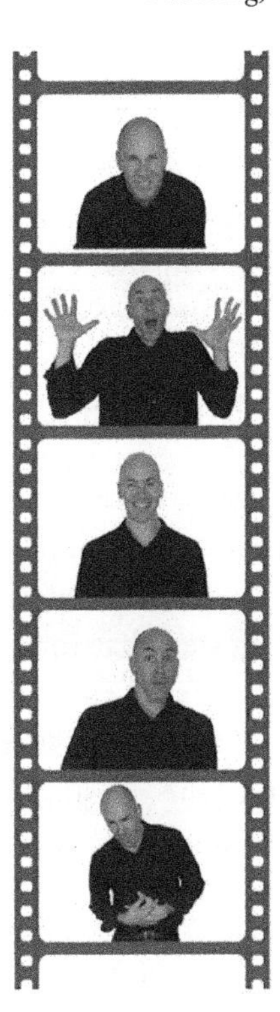

Figure 6.5: Different emotional expressions

more sensitive a nurse is in detecting the emotions of patients, the better able he or she will be in intervening or even in preventing problems. If a nurse can detect annoyance (see Figure 6.4.) in a patient, it will be possible to do something about it before it moves up the intensity scale and turns into anger or rage.

Through our behaviours and facial expressions we communicate our emotions to others. It is essential within any group, family or community that the members are aware of each other's emotions, because this gives us an opportunity to respond effectively. Ekman and Friesen performed a series of studies in different cultures in which they used photographs of faces that expressed a variety of emotions (See Figure 6.5.) (Ekman and Friesen, 1971; Ekman *et al.*, 1987). They found that there was considerable agreement in the judgement of these emotions across cultures. Like Plutchik, they concluded that we are most likely to be biologically prepared not only to experience but also to express and reliably recognise basic emotions in others. This quality is essential for the provision of good care by nurses.

Emotional labour

The efforts nurses put into reading and understanding patients' emotions are often identified as emotional labour (Gray, 2012). While it is important to develop this skill it can also be quite tiring. In a way, as part of understanding someone else's emotions, we tend to feel them ourselves to a certain extent. How much we feel depends on how close we are to the other. This is often considered the core of empathy and compassion. For instance, parents tend to feel more of their children's pains and joys than a stranger would. They often mention the burden that this puts on them. Similarly, for nurses, the burden of emotional labour and empathising with patients is an important issue (Kelly and Smith, 2016; Gray, 2012). It would seem that by not empathising enough we may be unable to respond effectively to patients' needs or provide a sense of rapport and trust. However, if we empathise without boundaries (in the way that parents often do with their children) we may put too much pressure on ourselves, which may lead to exhaustion (Selye, 1956) or burnout (Leiter and Maslach, 2009; Maslach *et al.*, 2001).

Emotions and thinking

In the past, much of emotion research and theorising focused on establishing the order of arousal, thinking and the actual emotion. William James (James, 1884) believed that we would experience arousal first and then interpret it according to cues in the environment. Cannon-Bard (Dror, 2014) suggested that these processes may take place simultaneously. Still others suggested that both arousal and emotion would take place after interpretation or appraisal of a situation (Lazarus and Folkman, 1984; Schachter and Singer, 1962). While the latter approach confirms common sense, the question remains: do we always have time to think or appraise? Perhaps we need to discriminate between fast and automated emotions, and less fast ones mediated by cognition. It is important for nurses to be aware of this distinction. To try and talk someone out of an emotion they have no conscious control over may be difficult. For instance, if you address a classically conditioned fear of blood by stating rational reasons not to be afraid, the person will say, 'I understand but still I panic'. Your approach may not help and you may also make the person feel stupid.

Case study: Emotional conditioning

Ali (58) has been in and out of hospital with cancer several times in the last year. He has undergone surgery and several other painful and uncomfortable treatments. His condition has been critical on a few occasions. He has been in Intensive Care and different wards in the hospital, and has been treated by several doctors and many nurses. When you have a conversation with him he says: 'It is strange, but every time I am here I feel increasingly sad and more and more sensitive. This hospital is really starting to push my buttons.' Consider which kind of events may have conditioned Ali to feel this way?

Complex emotions

In addition to primary emotions such as disgust, fear and surprise there are also more complex emotional states. First and foremost, we may experience more than one primary emotion at the same time. We may, for instance, feel grief and anger in response to the death of someone. Or we may feel amazement, joy and admiration when we see a well-performed circus act. When emotions are mixed together, it is often less easy to identify or communicate exactly what we feel. Secondly, there are complex states of feeling such as shame, guilt and embarrassment (Tangney and Fisher, 1995) that occur primarily when we are experiencing internal conflict (see the final section of this chapter). Some researchers consider **secondary emotions** (empathy, shame, pride, grief, guilt, jealousy, and embarrassment) (Konok *et al.*, 2015; Lewis, 2002) as equally universal as primary emotions. There are also debates around whether drive-like states such as lust, loneliness, ambition, hunger, thirst or pain should be classified as emotions or as motivation. Finally, there are moods that linger over time such as elation, wellbeing or depression that muddy our clarity on exactly what classifies as an emotion and what does not.

Moods

In comparison with emotions, moods tend to be more diffuse and linger longer. We mostly distinguish between upbeat (confident, optimistic, carefree, etc.) and low moods (pessimistic, powerless, vigilant, anxious, self-conscious, etc.). Moods reflect endocrine and neural activations that either energise or reduce energy levels and enhance or reduce access to pleasure or pain sensations. When people are already in an agitated mood and sympathetically aroused, emotions such as anger are felt more intensely. Moods also colour our perceptions and our memories of events. The 'mood congruency effect' (Bower, 1981) suggests that we are more prone to remember events that fit our mood (Fiedler *et al.*, 2001). Studies have shown that low mood reduces self-expectations (Kanter *et al.*, 2015) and expectations of the beneficence of social situations (Bower, 1991). Interestingly enough, a study on induced sadness showed that low moods could be countered by actively recalling positive memories (Josephson, 1996). Since patients in hospitals may not have the means to positively control their moods as they do at home, they may need this kind of support from nurses. The active induction of positive mood and optimism deserves the effort on the part of hospital staff. Research on the **mood contagion effect** (Neumann and Strack, 2000) confirms what most nurses already know: that whether they are upbeat or downbeat affects their patients likewise. With depression currently the most disabling disorder worldwide, in terms of premature mortality and years of disability (Whiteford *et al.*, 2013), it makes sense for nurses to become aware of what they can do to affect low mood in patients. We'll come back to this in Chapter 8.

Consistency and inconsistency in thinking, motivation, feelings and action

We tend to act in a smooth fashion when motivation, thinking and emotions line up in a consistent manner. Consistency allows us to operate efficiently and with a sense of flow.

However, often **inner conflicts** interrupt this smooth manner of operation. We may struggle with conflicting motivations, mixed emotions, discrepancies in our thinking, or actions that are inconsistent with values or expectations. Considering the complexity of health care and the likelihood that things do not go according to plan, it is important to keep in mind that smooth operation may not be as common as we would like and we will often be dealing with moments in which our peace of mind is disrupted.

Let us look at this in more detail now, using three different nursing activities as examples (see Table 6.2).

Table 6.2: The relationship between thinking, motivation, feeling, and doing

Event	Activities	Motivation	Cognitions	Emotions	Possible complication/ inconsistency
Discussion of diagnosis with patient	Communication; person-centred care; answering questions.	Demonstrate communication skills; show care.	Understanding diagnosis; understanding patient.	Concern; compassion; empathy.	Diagnosis not accepted by patient or self.
Listening to grieving family member	Listening; showing empathy and compassion.	Provide effective emotional care.	Understanding emotional needs; reflection on making a human connection.	Empathy; compassion; resonate with grief.	Association with own memories of loss too strong.
Performing CPR	Fast and efficient operation; monitoring handling of patient.	Saving a life; perform to best ability.	Understanding correct performance of procedure; thinking about success/failure; use calming thoughts.	Fear; afterwards joy (if successful).	CPR fails; CPR succeeds but patient outcome is negative.

The discussion of a diagnosis with a patient will most likely go smoothly if communication is effective, questions are answered, and the nurse is motivated to get it right, understands the diagnosis and the patient, and is able to feel empathy and show compassion. If the diagnosis is hard to take for the patient, the demonstration of empathy will be vital. It will have been helpful to anticipate the possible reaction of the patient and consider how to respond. Complications are likely to emerge if the patient or the nurse believes the diagnosis is incorrect. The patient may become highly upset, which will require additional attention. If the nurse has issues with the diagnosis this will lead to discomfort, which is bound to linger. Transmitting a message we don't believe leads to inner conflict.

Listening to grieving family members requires a calm response, listening and showing empathy. Being motivated to provide emotional care, understanding emotional needs, feeling empathy and the ability to resonate with grief will make for a positive experience even in dark moments. It becomes hard if the nurse feels over-burdened. Someone else's grief has a tendency to trigger our own sorrow. If this happens, the nurse might feel conflicted about continuing the communication.

Activities performed under stress, such as CPR, need to be well-learned and practised to secure a degree of automatism. Also, the motivation to save someone's life is a big responsibility, perhaps too big to control arousal levels, therefore we will most likely see experienced nurses be driven by the more modest motivation to perform the task as well as possible. Cognitions should be focused on the activity, but worries about possible failure to save the person's life might well intrude. Calming thoughts may be necessary to dispel those intrusions if they interfere. Emotions during the process will most likely be suppressed because fear may be unhelpful. Emotions afterwards will depend on the outcome. Unsuccessful CPR has the potential to lead to self-blame as a typical manifestation of inner conflict around failure. This state is epitomised by inner turmoil around thoughts such as 'Could I not have done more?'

Concept summary: Cognitive dissonance and inner conflict

Cognitive dissonance theory (Festinger, 1957) deals with how we experience and respond to inconsistencies within our thinking and between behaviour and thinking. When we become aware of inconsistencies we experience discomfort or dissonance. This motivates efforts to reduce it and regain consistency by adapting our attitudes, perceptions, or behaviours until consistency and our peace of mind are restored. Mild dissonance may be felt as an annoyance, but strong dissonance can take the form of embarrassment, shame, regret, or anger with oneself. We might say, 'I have mixed emotions', 'I am acting against my better judgement', or 'I am between a rock and a hard place'. Dissonance is an important aspect of our functioning and understanding it is essential for nurses. Can you identify the core of the internal conflict in each of the three examples in Table 6.2 after the complications emerge? Also, can you make suggestions to reduce dissonance in each situation?

An outline answer is provided at the end of the chapter.

In conclusion, we've established that motivation, emotions and thinking interact and, because the processes are intertwined, it is often hard to keep them apart. These intimate interactions promote internal consistency and smooth action. Nonetheless, we often experience contradictions, inconsistencies and discrepancies. This can be a source of inner conflict and turmoil.

Chapter summary

- We have the ability to think in highly sophisticated and rational ways (Rational Wonder), but also in imprecise and stereotypical ways (Cognitive Miser). The latter is a risk factor in nursing.
- We are better at solving most problems when our sympathetic arousal is under control. Over-arousal becomes a problem when we have to address particularly difficult problems.
- Positive thinking is an important asset in health care.
- It is hard to see how you can be a nurse without a strong intrinsic motivation.
- Drive reduction theory and the Hierarchy of Needs provide a useful way of understanding motivational processes.

continued . . .

continued . . .

- Understanding your own emotions and those of your patients is a core element in good care. If you fail to find the right balance in your 'emotional labour' you may risk exhausting yourself.
- Cognition, emotions and behaviour may be consistent or inconsistent. Inconsistency feels unpleasant and motivates efforts to restore it.

Activities: brief outline answers

Scenario: Rational wonder and cognitive miser in nursing (see page 94)

After a day in which you've functioned partly in cognitive miser mode you may feel dissatisfied and unfulfilled. If this has become the routine, it may not bother you. That would be worrying.

Activity 6.1: Critical thinking (see page 95)

1) Cognitive Miser, 2) Rational Wonder, 3) Cognitive Miser, 4) Cognitive Miser, 5) Rational Wonder, 6) Cognitive Miser, 7) Rational Wonder, 8) Rational Wonder, 9) Rational Wonder, 10) Cognitive Miser.

Scenarios: Creative problem solving (see page 98)

Harry is making use of the principle that many conflicts can be resolved if the parties can be helped to see a solution as a win-win situation. Siobhan's solution avoids 'mindless' mistakes due to misreading similar names of medication. Storing by category ensures more contrast in medicine adjacent on the same shelf.

Scenario: Nurse motivation (see page 99)

Bukola shows intrinsic motivation while Rita demonstrates extrinsic motivation.

Scenario: New purpose-built psychiatric unit (see page 102)

Management would have reasoned that if staff were overly concerned with physical needs, safety and security, they may have found it difficult to focus on higher order motivation towards their work. Care levels would most likely be negatively affected by this.

Activity 6.2: Reflection on basic emotions (see page 104)

It is important to be aware of your emotions and what your strengths and limitations are in how you cope with and control your emotions. Developing emotional intelligence (EQ) is indispensable for nurses.

Concept summary: Cognitive dissonance and inner conflict (see page 109)

In each of the examples dissonance can emerge and be reduced in multiple ways. For instance, *diagnosis example*: communicating something you don't believe in is inconsistent with seeing yourself as honest. Dissonance reduction could take place if you change your mind about the diagnosis or openly contest the diagnosis. *Grief example*: not wanting to listen any more is inconsistent with being an empathetic nurse. Dissonance reduction is hard, staying and sharing your feelings may help. *CPR example*: failure is inconsistent with seeing yourself as a successful professional. Dissonance reduction will follow from emphasising that you've done all you could do and followed the correct procedure.

Further reading

Kahneman, D. (2011) *Thinking, fast and slow.* London, UK: Penguin.

This is a highly popular, evocative and accessible book on thinking in all its facets, warts and all.

Weiten, W. (2008) *Psyk.Trek 3.1: a multimedia introduction to psychology* (3rd Ed.). New York, NY: Wadsworth.

CD-ROM (or online access) provides an enjoyable introduction to psychology with splendid modules on cognition, problem solving, motivation and emotions.

Allan, H., Traynor, M., Kelly, D. and Smith, P. (Eds.) (2016) *Understanding sociology in nursing.* London, UK: Sage.

This sociological text provides a useful perspective on emotions in care. Chapter 5 is particularly relevant.

Useful websites

http://creativethinking.net/exercises

Creative Thinking is one of the many websites that gives you opportunities to do exercises to practise thinking skills.

https://www.mindtools.com/

Mind Tools Club website provides interesting tools for problem solving, strategising and other skills that are useful in business but also in health care.

https://www.youtube.com/watch?v=PJrh99A5oaI

An hour-long webinar on *Emotional Intelligence in Healthcare* (2014) with rich content on emotional intelligence for nurses.

https://www.youtube.com/watch?v=n6MRsGwyMuQ

Emotional Intelligence by Daniel Goleman – an animated book summary. In seven minutes you are presented with all core ideas in Goleman's influential book.

Chapter 7
We are social animals

Chapter aims

After reading this chapter you will be able to:

- understand and apply principles of social interaction to nursing and health care;
- describe how people respond to social influence and apply this to nursing and health care;
- recognise the powerful impact of situations on our behaviour, thinking and emotions and identify when this could become a problem;
- understand organisational and safety culture in health care.

Health care mostly takes place in a social context and nursing is an endeavour in which social interaction and influence are paramount. Hence, in this chapter we look at social interaction, starting with the core mechanisms of reciprocity, group dynamics, prejudice and bias, followed by a section on social influence highlighting conformity, obedience, role behaviour, and helping behaviour. The last sections in this chapter examine organisational and safety culture. Each of these topics is addressed with reference to health care and nursing.

Introduction

We are social animals (Aronson, 2004). This is a profound statement. It suggests that we are like other animals and that we should understand our social inclinations as similar to theirs. For instance, we may start crossing at a red pedestrian light when two or three other people do so. Just like sheep or cows do when they pass an obstacle. Or we may be obsequious or rebellious to an authority figure at work in the same way that most mammals show such behaviours when approaching an animal that is higher in the pecking order. Also, we may bond, support and be loyal to others within, but not so much outside, our social group in the same way as other mammals, in particular primates.

We respond in these ways often without deciding to do so. This is because, just like in animals, nature seems to have programmed us in these ways. Moreover, the social situations in which we find ourselves frequently tend to control us, rather than the other way around. This is the cornerstone of our understanding of social influence. In this chapter we will introduce and guide you towards empirical research that supports this and we will provide you with considerable insight in what you might expect from yourself and others when in the grip of a powerful social situation such as a hospital or other health-care setting.

Mechanisms in social interaction

Reciprocity

Why do we live and work in communities? Why do we spend time socialising with others for entertainment and relaxation? Why do we seek and give support to each other? The answer to all of these questions is simple: because, in general, being part of a community benefits us. A rule of thumb about community is: **there is no community without reciprocal activity**. This rule also applies to health care and it is essential that you are aware of it. I scratch your back, you scratch mine. I do you a favour, you do me a favour. I say hello to you, I expect you to say hello to me. Any favour you bestow on others is a social or work investment and the expectation is that there will be a return (Cialdini *et al.*, 1975).

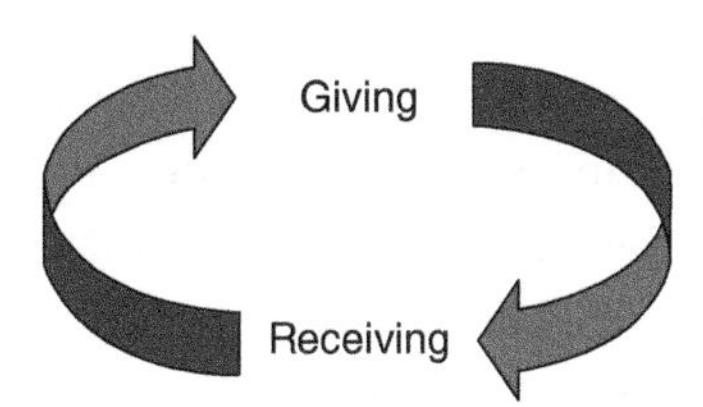

Figure 7.1: Reciprocity

Sometimes we expect reciprocity immediately, such as when we say hello. At other times a return of a favour can take place at some point later in time. An intricate network of favours and indebtedness generates the constant flurry of activity and movement in social and work relations. In general, we keep track rather well of who owes who. It is important that we do, because the social fabric would be undermined if we let cheaters (who don't return favours) off the hook (Cosmides and Tooby, 1992).

If we **trust** others and are in a constant exchange of favours, we are less concerned about the immediate return of the favour and reciprocal **altruism** (Trivers, 2006) may become the norm. This means that giving to others and receiving back something in return will be under less acute scrutiny. Under these conditions people will collaborate more effectively and trust each other more. Trust between people is a very important issue with a neurological and hormonal basis. It is hard to build, easily broken and hard to rebuild when broken (Kosfeld, 2007).

In your work as a nurse 'giving' in terms of energy and time and helping others is expected. You also expect to receive a return. Your wages are one form of return but, without harmonious work relationships and with a lack of reciprocal favours between colleagues, there may be trouble. In such cases it becomes necessary to look at which actions are not responded to as expected (see Table 7.1). We often underestimate how important it is to look at whether promises have been broken or whether there are other reasons for mistrust.

Table 7.1: Reciprocation in action

Action	Expected response
Do someone a favour	Favour acknowledged or returned
Something borrowed	Item returned
Greeting	Greeting in return
Work	Reasonable payment
Crime	Justice, restoration
Promise	Make good on promise
Pay health insurance premium	Receive good health care
Help and support patients	Recovery

In your relations with patients or clients the nurse is generally the one who is 'giving'. While the patient may expect your support (after all they need your help and they have paid for it in one way or form), they will still feel the need to reciprocate kindness and any help they perceive as beyond the call of duty. While limited in their ability to reciprocate, patients will nonetheless produce a smile, a friendly greeting or an expression of gratitude or appreciation. On top of this it could be argued that 'getting better' may be the most powerful way in which patients can repay your efforts.

Group formation, collaboration and competition

Reciprocation and altruism take place freely in established groups. Such groups are traditionally rooted in kinship. People in extended families support each other because they are thus benefiting those with genetic similarity (Gaulin and McBurney, 2001). This promotes **collaboration** and sharing with anyone we see as close to us. In contrast it is essential to appreciate that we are also hard-wired for **competition**. Like collaboration, competition is also an evolved adaptation (Flinn *et al.*, 2005; Buss, 1999) and is a core feature of how we live, mate and do business. Competition tends to become more evident when resources are limited and when observed differences between those competing are more obvious; think of ethnic and religious background, social class, language, professional background and political beliefs to name a few examples. These salient differences put us in groups that we may remain connected to throughout our lives, whether we want it or not. Membership of other groups can be more temporary and voluntary. A study group is a good example. We belong to many groups during our lives. These groups overlap and there are groups within groups. Within health care different professional groups, but also the distinction between care giver and care receiver, are subject to in-group/out-group mechanisms.

Activity 7.1 *Reflection*

Think about different professions and groups in a care organisation you know. List them and write them down. Consider the interactions between the groups and power differences. Use your experiences to identify the extent of collaboration, reciprocity and competition.

An outline response is provided at the end of the chapter.

We tend to accentuate collaboration within a group and competition between groups. However, we also often compete within groups (Buss, 1999). Often this presents itself in confusing ways. Children within a family may be extremely competitive, showing sibling rivalry but, at the same time, also showing collaboration (Goldenthal, 2000; Hudson and Trillmich, 2008). Play prepares them for both ways of interacting in the world. The hierarchical organisation within many groups promotes competition to move up in the pecking order while, at the same time, cooperation takes place. The formation of **coalitions** is a common sign of collaboration within an also competitive environment. Work 'friendships' are a good example of this. All workplaces, care organisations included, need these coalitions. They are like oil in an engine. In an environment that is too competitive these coalitions break down. Often this will be to the detriment of the overall effectiveness of work relationships and therefore the output of the organisation. Collaboration includes teamwork, sharing, cooperation, coordination and several other features that are essential to the functioning of organisations (Bedwell *et al.*, 2012). Collaboration cannot be taken for granted because we are so prepared for competition (see Table 7.2).

Table 7.2: Within and between-group (ingroup/outgroup) tendencies

Within-group tendencies	Between-group tendencies
Collaboration	Competition
Sharing of resources	Competition over resources
Helping and altruism	Bystander apathy and withholding help
Harmony	Conflict
Appreciating the unique person	Stereotyping, prejudice
Humanising	De-humanising

A famous reality experiment with teenage boys in an American summer camp showed how easy it was to create intense competition. In a matter of days, camp leaders succeeded in creating deep divisions between two arbitrarily generated equal-sized groups. All tendencies described in Table 7.2. became apparent. Artificially created status differences and competitive games led to stereotyping and prejudice. Interestingly, once the division had deepened, opportunities to intermingle were no longer used for friendly interactions, but for name calling and other prejudicial behaviour. Only by generating an overarching need for collaboration could the competition between the two groups be overcome (Sherif *et al.*, 1961). Similar findings in education also point at the importance of common goals in which all have to collaborate to succeed as the core to overcoming group divisions (Aronson and Bridgeman, 1992). Perhaps you've experienced how you were playing a ball game in which you were fiercely competitive, until the ball got lost in the bushes and you had to work together to get it out.

Within health care, the different professional groups sometimes behave in competitive ways. Different status, different uniforms and other symbols accentuate this. The social psychological literature suggests that collaboration as equals with the need for the help of all involved can break through divisions (Aronson, 2004; Aronson and Bridgeman, 1992). Extrapolating from this, we might be able to unite the professions in shared purpose and quest. The call for the development of shared **interdisciplinary** teaching at universities is a step aimed at overcoming these problems. Close collaboration in multi-disciplinary teams is another step, which is a common feature of modern health-care practice. However, more needs to be done because, as we've seen, closer contact by itself will not solve the problem if no effort is made to accentuate the need for each other's contribution in collaboration and the bringing about of more egalitarian interactions.

Scenario: Mental health care in the community

Mental health care in the community in the city was pretty much segregated along racial and ethnic lines. Each community mental-health team consisted only of people of one ethnic background that seemed to cater for its 'own people'. There was racial tension in the neighbourhoods and also between the mental-health teams. Resulting from a funding deficit, several of the teams were dismantled and the best-qualified staff were reallocated. This meant desegregation of the teams and also, for the first time, clients were going to meet with a nurse from a different ethnic background. The management team decided to set up interracial mental-health nursing buddy teams to make the transition and provide the introductions. Work was organised in such a way that collaboration was necessary and a less hierarchical team structure was created. Which elements in this change management plan might be instrumental to a successful transition?

An outline response is provided at the end of the chapter.

Between-group tendencies also exist between health-care professionals and those who receive care – the patients, clients or service users. This issue was flagged long ago by Lorber (1975) who highlighted that patients are often treated as the out-group by staff, particularly if they are seen as difficult or problem patients. This has a negative effect on the therapeutic relationship and can lead to compromised care levels and even abuse. It is sad to see that, in particular, vulnerable groups such as mental-health patients, people with intellectual disabilities, and elderly people suffering from dementia are at risk (Care, 2012; Phelvin, 2014). An important factor that brings out abusive behaviours is the **dehumanisation** of clients or patients. Once we accept treatment of patients that is undignified we are on our way to dehumanising them. We come back to this in Chapter 10.

Prejudice

It is perhaps a shock to have to admit to yourself that you are inherently prejudiced. The Museum of Tolerance in Los Angeles makes this point to all its visitors. After having bought a ticket there is a choice of two doors to enter the museum. One door is for prejudiced people, the other for the non-prejudiced. If you attempt to enter using the unprejudiced door it turns out that it is locked and a sign lights up saying 'Think ... Now, Use Other Door'.

Concept summary: The evolution of prejudice

Social psychological studies have demonstrated how easily we activate prejudice and stereotypes. Evolutionary psychology gives us the reasons for this. Firstly, our brain may have evolved preparedness for prejudice or stigmatisation against the old, vulnerable and infirm, motivating avoidance and exclusionary behaviour against them. This may have been adaptive in ancient times when resources to feed the community were limited. It may also have protected hunter-gatherers from contracting transmittable diseases. Secondly, evolutionary psychologists would argue for the adaptiveness of simplistic ways of understanding our social world in terms of who is within or outside our group and who is friend or foe. Our ancestor hunter-gatherers would have benefited from activating the concept 'different from us and dangerous' automatically and instantly when encountering someone from another tribe. Raiding other tribes was common practice so the assumption of animosity will have helped our ancestors survive by being quick enough to strike the first blow or getting out of the way quickly.

In nursing we encounter colleagues and people in our care who are ethnically or racially different, speak another language, or are otherwise different. We must therefore learn to override our prejudices and embrace diversity. Even so, when we feel insecure, threatened, angry, wound up, overwhelmed, stressed, hurried or tired we may still activate these fundamental tendencies (Fiske, 2004; Fiske, 2000) and act on them (see 'Cognitive Miser' approach in Chapter 6). That this can be a problem is well documented in research on stereotyping and prejudice against patient groups by health-care professionals (Ross and Goldner, 2009; Eliason, 1993). In turn, prejudices in general society affect nurses, particularly when they work in the community. Working with people with illnesses such as HIV-AIDS, physical handicaps, mental-health problems and intellectual disabilities often make us acutely aware of the stigma they experience (see also the section on Stigma in Chapter 9). This can sometimes be a significant obstacle to providing care and support in the community. It is essential to understand this within the context of in-group/out-group mechanisms and inherited tendencies to stereotype.

Scenario: Towards community integration

Jennifer is an intellectual disability nurse who works in a residential setting with 12 people with a moderate ID. The community housing project consists of three adjacent units in a neighbourhood with mainly families with children in the commuter belt of a major city. The people in Jennifer's care are not well accepted in the neighbourhood and, while they go shopping and visit a local community centre, there is virtually no interaction with the families in the area. Jennifer would like to do something about this. Using principles addressed in this chapter so far, how would you advise Jennifer?

An outline response is provided at the end of the chapter.

A jungle of bias

As we've already outlined in the Cognitive Miser approach to thinking (see Chapter 6), people often use biased thinking. We are subject to the halo effect, false-consensus effect, illusory correlation, confirmation bias, hindsight bias, fundamental attribution error, actor-observer bias, egocentric thought, self-serving bias, group think decoy, contrast effect, priming, framing, primacy effect, attention decrement, dilution effect, representative heuristic, availability heuristic and attitude heuristic, to name a few. It would go too far to go through all of them, but we'll address a few that are of particular relevance to nursing.

An essential bias to be aware of is called **actor-spectator bias** (Jones and Nisbett, 1971). This bias affects, for instance, how we attribute causes for a patient's annoyance to a problematic nature, instead of scrutinising the circumstances that may lead to the anger. If we were angry ourselves we would be quick to point out the external reasons for it, but in others we often fail to see them. There is a whole slew of publications highlighting the problems generated by 'the difficult patient' (Peterson, 1967; O'Sullivan, 2015; Sykes and Javidnia, 2013) which is rooted in this bias.

Another important challenge for nurses is **confirmation bias**, the principle that we tend to look for confirmation rather than falsification of what we currently believe (Aronson, 2004; Wason and Johnson-Laird, 1972). This can be to our detriment and even dangerous because it may cloud our judgement in a wide variety of situations. For instance, after a diagnosis has been made we tend to look for additional evidence to support it rather than being equally perceptive of counter indications. Another example is that once a treatment has been started, we are more likely to emphasise its benefits and we are at risk of ignoring signs of possible harm. This bias is one of the main reasons why mistakes are generally not recognised when the first signs appear. Interestingly enough, once a mistake has been recognised, with hindsight we start to see all those signals that we initially more or less ignored because they now confirm the altered perspective on the diagnosis or treatment. We call this **hindsight bias**.

We see the principle of confirmation also affect how we judge people and situations. The information that reaches us first generates **priming** or a 'frame of mind' that we then expand on in the assessment of further information. So, your first impression of a colleague or patient may colour your further judgement.

Activity 7.2 *Evidence-based practice and research*

Framing or priming

Which colleague do you like most? Explain the mechanism of bias.

- Nurse X, who is intelligent, industrious, impulsive, critical, stubborn and envious.
- Nurse Y, who is envious, stubborn, critical, impulsive, industrious and intelligent.

An outline response is provided at the end of the chapter.

Of course you will realise that the qualities are the same, only the order is different. Regardless, if you are like most people, you may find it hard to like Nurse Y as much as Nurse X. The positive qualities when read first tend to affect how we assess the more negative ones that follow and vice versa (Asch, 1946).

Also, for some reason, we tend to favour people who are considered **attractive** (Dion *et al.*, 1972; Berscheid and Walster, 1974). We tend to be nicer to attractive people, more prepared to give them the benefit of the doubt and find it harder to believe that they have engaged in crime or misdemeanour (Aronson, 2004). Attractive people are favoured in a court of law (Fraga, 2015), as employees (Hosoda *et al.*, 2003) and do not get fired as easily (Commisso and Finkelstein, 2012). Whether or not attractive patients get better treatment is an uncomfortable question. While no specific research seems to have been done on this issue, accumulated bias, including low attractiveness, has been shown to have a negative impact on a helper's perspective of patients (Wills, 1978).

Finally, in nursing, we sometimes stereotype ourselves. If we do so in negative ways, this may have an adverse impact on our performance. Studies on **stereotype threat** have demonstrated that the task performance of several ethnic and professional groups was negatively affected if a stereotype around such groups was reinforced just before the performance of the task (Walton *et al.*, 2015; Steele *et al.*, 2002). Thus, when African-Americans were told that a mathematics task they were about to engage in was not usually done as well by African-Americans as by Asian-American participants, they performed less well than they normally did (Steele and Aronson, 1995). If they did not receive this information as part of the instructions, this effect did not take place. Similar studies have demonstrated that stereotype threat also affects gender differences (Davies *et al.*, 2005; Spencer *et al.*, 1999). Do the stereotypical beliefs nurses have about themselves affect performance? Think about it (see Chapter 10). What do you think these stereotypes are? Budding research on this issue suggests that public perspectives of nursing can affect nursing performance (Takase *et al.*, 2006).

Activity 7.3 — *Critical thinking*

Identify the types of bias you see here:

- You have just been in the ICU nursing very frail people. You find yourself seeing other patients as more vulnerable.
- You consider a 16-year old boy who is scared of going to the toilet by himself a wimp (until you hear that an attack in a toilet was the reason he is in hospital).
- A doctor tells you that most nurses do not understand the brain very well. After this you find yourself unable to have a conversation about the brain.
- A patient diagnosed with cancer was treated for a whole year as if she was severely ill, until finally a second opinion contradicted the diagnosis.
- You notice that a patient with a disfigurement does not receive the same smile that her attractive neighbour gets.

An outline answer is provided at the end of the chapter.

Social influence

Research on social influence has been a headline grabber in social psychology. Studies on **conformity, obedience, role behaviour and bystander apathy** have had a strong impact on how we understand ourselves and, although the original studies were done between 1955–1975, they still speak to us and recent replications have more or less produced the same findings. Nurses will learn a lot about these topics by completing Activity 7.4 and looking up the revealing video footage that is available online. We will focus on the application of each of these topics to nursing and health care in this section.

Activity 7.4 *Evidence-based practice and research*

Fact finding mission: look up online (YouTube, Wikipedia), discuss and answer the following questions.

Describe **Solomon Asch's** famous study on conformity. What were the main findings? Why should the outcomes concern health-care staff?	Describe **Stanley Milgram's** famous study on obedience. What were the main findings? Why are the outcomes important to health-care staff?
Describe **the Stanford Prison Study (Zimbardo, Haney, Prescott)**. What were the main findings? Why are the outcomes of interest in health care?	Describe **Latané and Darley's** work on bystander apathy. What were the main findings? How can nurses prevent bystander apathy?

Conformity

Conformity exhibits itself in uniform behaviour without obvious pressure other than that others are observed as behaving in the same way. It is helpful for the smooth running of health-care institutions or any complex organisation or business if conformity is high. However, research on conformity also highlights its undesirable side. A famous study by Solomon Asch (1956) demonstrated that, under the pressure of a group making obviously wrong decisions, individuals were highly likely to conform and make the same wrong decision. The impact of conformity is such that we feel extremely uncomfortable if we are seen as different from everybody else and, even if we know we are wrong, we are prepared to do as everybody else does. This has been demonstrated to be a problem in health care. Whenever a majority demonstrates substandard or incorrect practice, it is likely that the rest of the staff will follow. To break ranks tends to be extremely difficult or stressful (Asch, 1956; Hodges and Geyer, 2006; Dungan *et al.*, 2015), especially when the whole organisation turns against the individual. Whistleblowers sometimes report having gone 'through hell' as part of their efforts to expose malpractice.

There is more to this, as research on group decision making shows that conformity, when combined with other mechanisms, can lead to highly suspect decisions. A combination of friendly relationships, strong opinion leaders and exclusionary behaviour against critical or different perspectives can lead to what is referred to as **group think** (Janis, 1982). Hospital boards and MDTs have sometimes been shown to be at risk of operating in this way and losing a critical perspective on their operations. It is important to note when things are getting too cushy and criticism or alternative perspectives get stifled.

Obedience

In most health-care organisations decisions are made and orders are given by management with authority at different levels. Obedience is needed to ensure that rules, regulations and directives are followed. On balance you might argue that, like conformity, obedience has more advantages than drawbacks. However, obedience also has a dark side, as Milgram's (1963) (in)famous studies demonstrated. His research showed that normal, well-intentioned people cast in the role of teachers instructed by an authority figure were prepared to give painful shocks to punish a learner when he made mistakes. The study was carefully choreographed and, while no actual shocks were received by the learner, everything was done to make the teacher believe the ploy.

At the time, Milgram's results were often questioned, but even recent replications (Burger, 2009) have demonstrated that they were no fluke. Milgram's original study only included male participants, but similar outcomes have been found with female participants. Milgram varied different aspects of the design in subsequent studies. Eventually this led him to conclude that obedience was highest when the authority was in close proximity to the participant, while the victim being hurt was in a different room. Recent replications emphasise that the extent to which participants identified with the authority or the victim made a difference. Obedience was highest when the first was high and the latter low (Haslam and Reicher, 2012). If we translate this to health care, we would predict nurses to be more obedient when under direct supervision. In cases of abusive treatment of patients, low levels of identification with their plight will have contributed to this.

Scenario: The obedient nurse

Melina is assisting with a procedure that is not performed as required. The consultant seems not to notice, which concerns her. The next day she helps with the same procedure with a different patient, and the same thing happens. Melina does not know what to do. She is trying to make sense of her indecision. Can you help her, using the principles addressed in this chapter?

An outline response is provided at the end of the chapter.

Role behaviour

Nurses in the General or Children's nursing discipline mostly wear a uniform. This is an important statement for the patient. Mental health and ID nurses don't. This is also an important statement to their clients or service users. Wearing a uniform seems to say, 'I am a professional and will perform according to uniform standards'. Not wearing a uniform is more like saying, 'In essence I am just like you and I will support you as an equal'. Each is appropriate for the different settings in which care is given.

Specific expectations come with the uniform. A person in a hospital in a white coat with a stethoscope around the neck will automatically be regarded as a doctor or nurse. Yet, expectations of ourselves are also affected when we put on the uniform. The uniform puts you in the nurse's role and this may affect how you perform. Ellen Langer's (Langer *et al.*, 2010) research with pilots in a flight simulator demonstrated that when they were wearing their uniforms and in their role as pilots this significantly improved their visual acuity. It is highly likely that if such a study was done with nursing students when performing typical nursing tasks we would also see higher perceptual acuity when in uniform and fully engaged in the nursing role. It would seem that adopting a professional role activates us in ways that would make us more effective in performing that role.

Sometimes roles can take on a total reality that makes us lose perspective and perform them without questioning them. This was demonstrated in the Stanford Prison Experiment (Zimbardo *et al.*, 1974). Students put in the roles of prisoners became passive or depressed and those in the role of guards developed a brutality that surprised all involved. There is much evidence in the world that this is reflective of reality in general. Even in hospitals we can see nurses and doctors who find themselves at risk of adopting a particularly controlling version of their role and they lose perspective of patients' needs. Conversely, we may identify patients who have adopted an overly passive version of the 'patient role' and they run the risk of becoming more helpless than is good for them.

Helping and bystander apathy

Normally we are inclined to help others when a direct appeal for our help is made. From an evolutionary perspective this makes sense because such appeals would most likely come from members of our community and it would have been adaptive to help as part of the system of reciprocation in which we lived (Buss, 1999). We would have expected to be helped in return. Empirical research on helping confirms this principle (Gross and Latané, 1974). Cognitive dissonance theory further explains the moral decision making around helping. We help because not helping violates our belief in ourselves as good people (Aronson, 1969) and generates 'dissonance discomfort'.

Notwithstanding this, and just like with several of the studies mentioned in the above, social psychological research on helping behaviour has provided us with very unflattering insights into human behavioural tendencies. Experiments done in public out on the street have demonstrated that ordinary people often fail to assist someone who seems unconscious or in need of medical attention (Latané and Darley, 1969; Darley and Latané, 1968; Latané and Nida, 1981). This is called **bystander apathy** and, contrary to what you might expect, it is stronger when more passive spectators are present. Of course when you, as a nurse, would appear on the scene you would most likely break through this apathy. Motivated by your professional ethos and relevant knowhow, you would help. This would change things, as research also demonstrated (Schwartz and Clausen, 1970; Cacioppo *et al.*, 1986). The upshot is that helpers can be recruited effectively once a person starts and engages others by addressing them in person with specific instructions ('You in the blue jacket, please come here and hold his head. You with the red scarf, do you have a mobile phone? Please call emergency services.'). Your professional role will give you authority ('I am a nurse, I need you to assist me now.'). Once people have accepted responsibility, they are highly likely to take this seriously (Aronson, 2004). Recent debate by nursing scholars on bystander apathy in nursing and health care (Paley, 2014; Darbyshire, 2014; Mannion and

Davies, 2015; Rydon-Grange, 2015) suggests that it is particularly important for nurses to remain vigilant.

Working in a large health-care organisation

We have looked so far at the mechanisms by which individuals, and specifically nurses, are affected in social and work situations. In addition, there are organisational aspects relevant to health care we would like to include to complete the picture. We will focus on two factors: organisational culture and safety culture.

Organisational culture

All organisations are imbued with ways of communicating, ethos, ideals, ways of doing business, ways of maintaining quality, beliefs and values, etc. We call this the organisational culture. It is expressed in brochures, standards and regulations but, more importantly, in informal ways. When you first start a placement, staff will communicate the organisational culture and its unspoken rules to you and initiate and socialise you into it. Of course there are moments when your ideas may clash with the culture of the hospital and you may be pulled aside to be told, 'that is not how we do things here'. Awareness of the organisational culture and its impact on your work is useful to ensure that you function in accordance with it, but also to be able to critically examine it.

Activity 7.5 *Critical thinking*

Study these organisational vignettes and discuss the questions at the bottom.

Organisation A	**Organisation B**
The work requires very little skill and limited knowledge. It is physically exhausting, unhealthy and monotonous. Staff tend to do as they are told. The work does not offer opportunities for individual initiative. The pay tends to be based on the extent of the availability of a potential unskilled labour force. Typically the company is not concerned when staff want to leave employment, as long as replacements can be hired instantly. Often not much is done to protect the staff or optimise working conditions. Career opportunities within the company are usually not available for the staff who do this work. They end up feeling that they only continue because they need the income.	The work requires skills and knowledge that can only be mastered after several years of education. While the work is physically hard and mentally exhausting, it requires a responsible attitude and the ability to take the initiative and to make important decisions. Experience is built up over time and so the value of staff increases over the years. While wages are not particularly high at the outset, they increase over time. A career path tends to be available to ensure that staff can keep developing and engage in 'self-actualisation' (see Chapter 6). Training opportunities and a philosophy of life-long learning go hand in hand in this development.

continued . . .

continued . . .

Discuss:

1. To what extent do you recognise nursing in the two models?
2. Discuss your own expectations with reference to models A and B.

An outline response is provided at the end of the chapter.

How an organisation relates to its staff is essential to its organisational culture. The more staff invest in terms of time, effort, education, etc., the more is expected in return. The idea that work is just an economic exchange in which the organisation is committed only to paying wages is becoming obsolete. In particular, health-care organisations are communities and they should facilitate social and health support, opportunities for development, and leisure activities. Contemporary perspectives emphasise the rationality of supporting the wellbeing of staff because it is in the interest of the smooth running of the organisation and the care of patients.

It is important to realise that the complexity of a health-care organisation and its size play an important role in its organisational culture. Large health-care organisations, such as most hospitals, tend to be run in hierarchical fashion with **top-down decision making**. This means that decisions are made by a small group at the top who communicate the orders down the hierarchy. Those at the bottom of the hierarchy usually have little say and, in its purest form, are only expected to execute the decisions. In smaller organisations, such as community health teams, we are more likely to see **bottom-up decision making** in which all have a degree of responsibility and decisions are made where the activities take place. Recent research supports personal responsibility as essential to productivity in health care (Biller-Andorno and Zeltner, 2015; Vargas and Ramos, 2011).

When organisations grow from small to large they often undergo a period of significant change in which the old way of working is replaced with new, more formal, structures. A word or two between colleagues becomes a meeting with an agenda and a chair. An informal checking of work practices becomes a documented auditing. This can be alienating, especially for staff with a long history within the organisation, and it requires well thought out **change management** (Hasegawa and Karandagoda, 2011). Many hospitals undergo radical changes in their infrastructure, size, and the way they work. Staff often find it difficult to adjust to these changes, which leads to increased stress levels (Murphy, 1996). In the long term, high stress levels among staff tend to come with increased health risks, increases in sick days, and eventually this will impact the quality of patient care (Leiter and Maslach, 2009; Maslach, 2003; Firth-Cozens and Greenhalgh, 1997). How an organisation deals with this is also part of its organisational culture.

Safety culture

Most organisations aim to optimise their output and minimise their costs. Most organisations also have to deal with risks and dangers. Safety is especially important in hospitals because there are many risks and patients and staff may die if safety procedures are not optimised. You may find it difficult to distinguish between health-care output and safety procedures because they are so intertwined. With almost every activity there are several accompanying safety measures. For every single injection you check the needle is sterile (1), check you are using the correct substance (2), check the use-by date (3), check the patient's chart (4), check with the patient that they are expecting the injection (5) you wash your hands (6) you consider whether you have perhaps forgotten something (7). Nonetheless mistakes are made. Reason warns that safety measures, while often developed over many years and geared towards dealing with many eventualities, generally look better on paper than they are in reality. He calls this the **Swiss Cheese** model of accidents (Reason *et al.*, 2006; Reason, 1990). If all holes or failings in the protective measures line up, an accident takes place.

Case study: Hospital safety

Health-care organisations are no different from manufacturing plants, airlines, building companies, software providers, oil refineries, etc. in that they work according to economic principles. These include controlling spending, limiting hospital stays, and by deploying only the necessary number of staff. This has the potential to happen at the expense of the safety aspect (Reason, 1993). Some people such as health and safety officers and infection control nurses are specifically appointed to keep the safety issue on the agenda. Their problem is that an absence of incidents tends to instil a false sense of security and complacency. Can you explain why an infection control nurse is campaigning for anonymous reporting of small accidents and near misses?

An outline response is provided at the end of the chapter.

Paradoxically, Reason also emphasises that 'accidents must happen'. Hopefully they happen without fatal consequences but they must happen and be noted because this ensures that the organisation remains alert and motivated to keep optimising safety measures. Reason warns that unless we make sure that all small accidents and 'near misses' are reported, we may lose perspective and will be increasingly at risk of a major catastrophe. A common scenario emerging from research on major catastrophes looks somewhat like what is displayed in Figure 7.2.

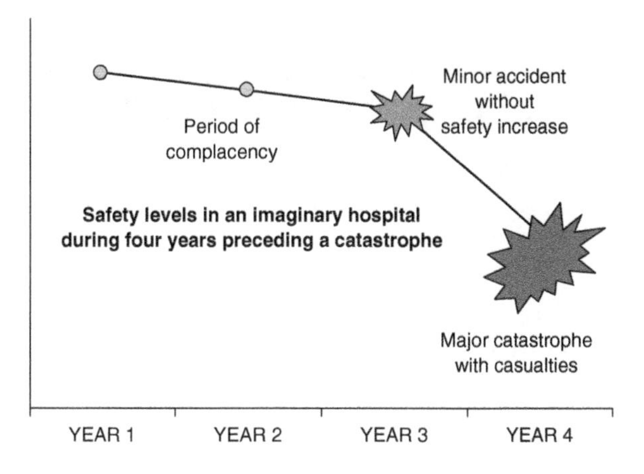

Figure 7.2: The impact of complacency and lack of response to minor accidents on safety leading to catastrophe (adapted from Reason, 1990)

Reason emphasises that it is a mistake to think that individual errors are the single cause of accidents. Most accidents have their origin in **structural hazards** (accidents waiting to happen). Small lettering on medication and bad light in the room where they are selected are examples of structural hazards that increase the risk of medication errors. Human error often merely activates the structural hazard. It is therefore the case that a positive safety culture should include reviewing, raising awareness, inviting reporting, and addressing of all structural hazards. This includes reconsidering unusually cumbersome safety measures that tend to invite violations. Nurses working within this force field need to be aware of how their organisation stands on safety culture and how this affects their own safety within the organisation. Awareness of the potential of the social mechanisms introduced in this chapter to affect the rational and safe operation of health-care organisations should be helpful in this respect.

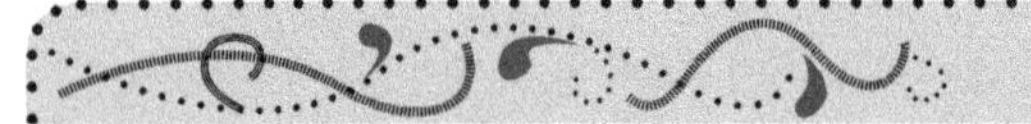

Chapter summary

- Awareness of the mechanisms of social interaction, social influence and the issues related to working in a large organisation is important. This will help you to recognise and promote desirable aspects and avoid the undesirable ones.
- Reciprocity is a guiding principle in maintaining good relationships with colleagues and people in your care.
- To be aware of our innate propensity to be prejudiced against those who are significantly different from us can help us to overcome this problem.
- There are many biases in our cognition that can be avoided by rational thinking.
- Human tendencies towards obedience and conformity can be very strong and may override our good judgement.
- Large health-care organisations have imposing organisational and safety cultures so it is important to identify how effective these cultures are in dealing with mistakes, accidents and near misses.

Activities: brief outline answers

Activity 7.1: Reflection (see page 114)

Most likely you will have reflected on how care assistants, nurses, nurse managers, doctors, consultants, administrative personnel, etc. form distinctive groups with specific in-group and out-group relationships.

Scenario: Mental health care in the community (see page 116)

The effective ingredients of the change process are the creation of buddy relationships in which reciprocal collaboration is hoped to take place. Through having goals that can only be achieved through collaboration, racial and ethnic differences may become less salient.

Scenario: Towards community integration (see page 117)

It may not be easy but the key to the integration of the ID residents is to generate some kind of activity that starts reciprocity in the relationship with the families. Giving something to the community would be a good idea. Perhaps the neighbourhood needs to be educated about the ID residents to dispel prejudice.

Activity 7.2: Framing or priming (see page 118)

We can't help but like Nurse X more, because each positive term affect how we receive the next one. For Nurse Y, the opposite is the case. We do not process personal features independently.

Activity 7.3: Identify the types of bias you see here (see page 119)

1) Frame of mind or priming; 2) actor-spectator bias; 3) stereotype threat; 4) confirmation bias; 5) attractiveness bias.

Activity 7.4: Look up on line (YouTube and Wikipedia), discuss and answer the following questions (see page 120)

To provide elaborate answers here would defeat the purpose of the exercise. The essence has been presented in the section on Social influence. Also see Useful websites below.

Scenario: The obedient nurse (see page 121)

Melina's indecision may be the result of her reluctance not to conform or obey. This most likely creates cognitive dissonance. How she resolves the situation will depend on what would best reduce the dissonance she experiences. It is a tricky situation.

Activity 7.5: Study the vignettes and discuss the questions at the bottom (see page 123)

Organisation B is most like contemporary nursing but some of it may be aspirational. Elements of Organisation A may be representative of nursing in the past or in primitive circumstances. Try to understand that how you perceive and respond in an organisation may affect the opportunities that open up for you.

Case study: Hospital safety (see page 125)

The infection control nurse is trying to ensure that important safety information is gathered. Normally staff are reluctant to come forward when they've had a near miss, fearing that they will be punished. Anonymous reporting would help in getting a more accurate picture of structural hazards.

Further reading

Aronson, E. (2004) *The social animal* (9th Ed.). New York: Worth.

This brilliant introduction to social psychology is comprehensive, eloquent and reads like a novel.

Reason, J. T. (1997) *Managing the risks of organisational accidents.* Aldershot, UK: Ashgate.

To further your understanding of organisational risk and safety this is essential reading.

Klein, W. M., Shepperd, J. A., Suls, J., Rothman, A. J. and Croyle, R. T. (2015) Realizing the promise of social psychology in improving public health. *Personality and Social Psychology Review,* Vol. 19(1): 77–92.

This article explores issues in public health with the use of social psychology.

Useful websites

http://www.learner.org/resources/series138.html

The famous *Discovering Psychology* series hosted by Prof. Philip Zimbardo, watch nr 19: 'The Power of the Situation'.

https://www.youtube.com/watch?v=EoU0Kbiw9RE

Social Psychology Behavior Lab Conformity. This video shows recent research on conformity, replications of Solomon Asch's work and more.

http://jfmueller.faculty.noctrl.edu/crow/helping.htm

Website with rich AV and written resources on Social Psychology, including sections on Helping and Altruism.

Chapter 8
The psychology of health and stress

Chapter aims

After reading this chapter you will be able to:

- apply the bio-psycho-social model in health care and nursing;
- discuss psychological aspects of core health factors such as nutrition and exercise;
- understand how our thinking about health is affected by principles of attribution, cognitive consistency, and self-protection;
- compare and apply several models of stress and stress management.

This chapter will provide an introduction to the psychology of health and stress. Health psychology is a relatively new but rapidly developing branch of psychology. This chapter will start with an introduction to this field and an exploration of the bio-psycho-social model in health and health care today. We continue by exploring the psychology of core factors in health such as nutrition and exercise. Following this we discuss how our thinking affects health related behaviour. The chapter is concluded with an overview of stress theories and their implications for health.

Activity 8.1 *Critical thinking*

A GP visit in 2050

A woman goes to her family doctor. The doctor asks her whether she has any complaints. 'On the contrary', she says, 'I just wanted to come and report that I have been feeling amazingly healthy and well recently'. She continues to explain that she would like to discuss how changes in her life may have contributed to this in order to pinpoint the essential factors with the help of an expert. She argues that this might then help her to ensure that she will more often be so healthy and feel so well.

The GP's reality now

The convention of doctor visits is that we are only supposed to go if we have a health problem or worry, if we need an inoculation or if we need a check-up. It has always been this way. We should, therefore, not be surprised that GPs (and other doctors) know much more about illness than about health. They are trained and experienced in interventions to address illnesses, somewhat adept at prevention of illness, but how to achieve great health is something that they do not really encounter in their practice.

continued . . .

continued . . .

1. **A GP visit in 2050**. Could this ever become a common GP visit? Debate a future for health care in which this GP visit would be a normal event.
2. **The GP's reality now**. Expand on today's GP consultations. What are GPs' strengths and limitations? What changes would be possible?

Some thoughts are provided at the end of the chapter.

The development of health psychology

Medical science has traditionally focussed on illness – its diagnosis, causes and cures. This is considered the core of the **bio-medical model** of health care. Little attention was devoted to illness prevention, how health can be maintained, and how psychological and social factors affect health and illness. However, in the last 50 years things have changed. Today we no longer believe health care should only concentrate on illness and we no longer believe that illness and loss of health only have physiological causes. In this new era, health care is veering towards more emphasis on achieving positive health and wellness. This includes developing an understanding of how illness can be prevented through a healthy life style and proactive use of medical services, and a variety of other factors in which awareness, attitudes and behaviours play a role.

Essential to this change are the newly developing fields of behavioural medicine and health psychology. Health psychology can be defined as 'an interdisciplinary field concerned with the application of psychological knowledge and techniques to health, illness and health care' (Marks *et al.*, 2011, p. 11). Behavioural medicine bridges the gap between medicine and psychology from the medical side. Emerging areas such as psycho-immunology, psycho-oncology and psycho-endocrinology are part of this development. Its foundation was laid in the 1970s and 1980s, with the challenge to the bio-medical model and the introduction of a new approach that included psychological and social factors – the **bio-psycho-social model** (see Ch. 1: Figure 1.2). The main differences between the two approaches are presented in Table 8.1.

The core of the bio-psycho-social model is the recognition of the influence on our health of the world we live in and our own behaviour. The empirical basis for this started emerging as early as the 1950s. A good example is research on heart disease in managers – an emerging concern in the business world at the time – which demonstrated that personality and behavioural factors were the most accurate predictors of high risk (Friedman and Rosenman, 1959). Over the years the research showed that at-risk managers tended to be more competitive, authoritarian, and more easily angered. They generated frequent conflict and did not plan so well. This was called **Type A personality or behaviour**. The implication of this finding was that, instead of costly medical interventions, we should focus on much cheaper behavioural change. Findings such as this got psychologists and medics talking. More recent research has demonstrated that a variety of behavioural and social factors may lead to heart disease, including lack of exercise, unhealthy diet and resulting obesity (Mozaffarian *et al.*, 2016). These factors are

Table 8.1: Differences between the bio-medical and bio-psycho-social models of health and illness

Bio-medical	Bio-psycho-social
• Mind and body function *separately* • Cause of illness is *biological* • Individual patients are *not responsible* • Treatment of illness = *physiological intervention* • Illness is treated by the *medical profession* • Health and illness are *qualitatively different* • Illness has psychological consequences *not causes* • Focus on *illness*	• Mind and body *interact* • Illness can be caused by *bio-psycho-social* factors • Patients are *responsible* and may be actively involved in the causes of illness • Treatment of the *whole person* • Patient is *part responsible* for healing • Health and illness *are a continuum* • Psychology can be part of *cause and effect* • Focus on illness and *wellness*

also recognised today as contributing to the increase in Type II diabetes in Western society (Ezzati and Riboli, 2013).

A different kind of confirmation of the importance of social and behavioural factors came from **historical research**. McKeown (1979) studied documents tracing the incidence of tuberculosis (TB) in Europe from 1500 onwards and these revealed that the decrease in TB-related mortality was neither significantly affected by the discovery of the tubercle bacillus nor the invention and manufacturing of penicillin. However, it could be effectively explained by well-documented gradual improvements in hygiene, sanitation, and the availability of uncontaminated nutrition and water. His findings challenged the assumption that improvements in health throughout history were the result of medical advances only (McKeown, 2014; McKeown, 1979).

The campaign to reduce the smoking of tobacco illustrates how, in addition to the bio-psycho-social aspects, economic and political factors also affect health. After decades in which half the world seemed to be happily puffing away, medical researchers established the relationship between lung cancer, heart disease and smoking. People were shocked and health-care professionals and policy makers concluded that the cost in terms of human suffering and health-care expenses was unacceptable. Together this motivated a **campaign against smoking**. Further research and political effort was needed to defeat the efforts of the tobacco industry to confuse the issue. Economic measures, including taxation, made smoking more and more expensive and started to become another deterrent. Finally, a tipping point was reached. By the time bans on smoking in public places started to appear, support for it outweighed the protests. Today we see significant reductions in smoking all over the Western world. It is particularly interesting to see that when a wide variety of measures is taken, a significant and rapid shift in health behaviour is possible. Very few people would have predicted that this development would only take a couple of decades. Psychologists are prone to highlight the power of social influence (see Chapter 7). If initially conformity got us all smoking, the 'contagion of non-smoking' got us to give it up. Let us hope that the newly introduced e-cigarette will not cause regression on this issue.

Activity 8.2 — Critical thinking

Mr Aziz (71) is recovering from a heart attack. He came over from Iraq last year with a heart condition and is now living in Britain with his family. He was in the army until his retirement. He has smoked most of his life. He has had an operation on his aorta and will be moved to a rehabilitation unit. The family have suggested that he could perhaps move home where they can support him. Mr Aziz is in strong agreement with this. Both consultant and nursing staff think that a rehabilitation centre will benefit Mr Aziz considerably.

Discuss the scenario using the bio-psycho-social model:

1. What are the biological/medical concerns?
2. What are the psychological concerns?
3. What are the social factors?
4. Could you imagine possible economic, political or religious/spiritual factors?

An outline answer is provided at the end of the chapter.

The high cost of the treatment of many illnesses increasingly provides an incentive to promote **prevention** or early intervention, with an emphasis on changing public opinion and behaviour in regard to specific risk factors. Similarly motivated efforts to address Type II diabetes and obesity through psychological, social, economic, political, and even religious or spiritual means, could be on the cards. Complex global health problems such as HIV-AIDS are now recognised worldwide as rooted in multiple factors including psychological resistance and religious objections to the use of prophylactics. However, economic factors are a common thread. Many commentators emphasise that it is 'poverty' that leads to HIV-AIDS and it is therefore by addressing poverty that we can address the pandemic (Fenton, 2004; Mufune, 2015).

To conclude, it is evident that health care has been taken out of its isolation as the exclusive territory of medical experts. Today, politicians, religious leaders, economists, food producers and retailers, sociologists and health psychologists are assuming joint responsibility and sit around the table with medics to discuss health locally and internationally in organisations such as the World Health Organization (WHO).

Concept summary

The World Health Organization (WHO) is a UN agency that plays an active role in promoting the 'attainment by all peoples of the highest possible level of health' (WHO, 2006, p. 2). Thus the organisation promotes health and health care all over the world. Its mission statement includes several important principles such as that 'health is a state of complete physical, mental and social well-being and not merely the absence of disease or infirmity' (WHO, 2006). This perspective is representative of contemporary views of health rooted in the bio-psycho-social model. The WHO acknowledges that health is a human right, that there is considerable health inequality across the world, and that health promotion is a global issue with local progress ultimately providing benefits for all. For nurses, the WHO is of particular importance to broaden the horizon on health priorities elsewhere in the world (for example, hunger), which are very different from what tends to worry us most in the Western world (for example, obesity). Also, the WHO has produced authoritative reports on issues such as mental health, stress, cancer, HIV-AIDS, and even hand washing. These provide essential reading for nurses.

Activity 8.3 *Critical thinking*

Use WHO sources to list and discuss major health risks in rich and in poor countries. Establish differences and similarities. Suggest behavioural, social, economic and political interventions for each health risk. Which aspects can you influence as a nurse?

Some thoughts are provided at the end of the chapter.

Core health factors and psychology

In the section above we have outlined the determinants of health and their complexity within the bio-psycho-social model. Because nutrition and exercise are the most essential factors affecting our health we focus on these aspects next.

Psychology of nutrition

Eating enough and in a varied way is an important benefit to health. Conversely, long periods of malnutrition and hunger have a lasting negative impact on health and mental health (Weinreb *et al.*, 2002). While hunger is of great concern globally, today's concerns in the Western world are about overeating and 'what' we eat that causes us harm. Ideas of what a healthy diet is have developed significantly in the last 50 years. As a result, most people are familiar with the 'food pyramid', the importance of vitamins, and the health benefits of fish oils, vegetables and fruits. Paradoxically, at the same time, our eating habits have become a major health risk. Milan Kundera the novelist expresses it very well through one of his characters as he sits down to eat in a restaurant: 'Don't tell my doctor, but I have my own conception of a diet. I strictly avoid all those foods I don't enjoy' (Kundera, 1996, p. 175). This hits at the core of the problem. Our food preferences do not match what is most healthy for us. We overeat on **fat, salt and sugar** because we like it so much. Dieticians, nutritionists and parents are often frustrated at how difficult it is to bolster the motivation to reduce fat, salt and sugar intake.

Evolutionary theorists suggest that our great appetite for these nutrients goes back to our hunter-gatherer ancestors in Palaeolithic times (100,000 to 40,000 years ago). The survival benefits of fat are that it can be stored in the body and accessed in lean times. Salt helps us restore the water balance in the body, and sugars in nature are normally found in ripe fruits which contain significant nutrients and are a marker for vitamins. A strong motivation to eat as much of it as possible will have given those with this propensity a higher chance of survival. Overeating these nutrients was not a risk factor then because of scarcity. The animals we hunted were nomadic and had little fat on them. Fruits are seasonal and only at their sweetest for a brief while. Salt is scarce in many areas on earth. All of this has changed. Animal husbandry has led to fatter animals and we have learned to manufacture salt and sugar, now without the health benefits of the other nutrients in fruit. Our strong liking of fat, salt and sugar has become a problem because it is no longer scarce. Our food industry plays into these preferences and it is increasingly hard to buy products without boosted fat, sugar or salt content, often at the expense of the nutritional value. Today we recognise the problem but we still find it hard to solve it because of the strength of our preferences. It would seem that to be healthy today means having the strength to suppress our hunter-gatherer preferences and studying what we eat.

The study of what we should and should not eat has mushroomed but the principles at the basis of **diets** differ, taking into account conflicting nutritional or ethical principles. This is not the place to comment on this in detail, but it is of psychological interest that most people find it hard to stick to regimented eating patterns such as a diet. Conflicting perspectives have turned dieting efforts into confusing experiences that are often abandoned when new information is acquired. Moreover, the strength of our cravings can be so intense that we are highly prone to ignore dietary restrictions. Yo-yo dieting is common among people trying to lose weight, which in fact adds to the health risks (Brownell and Rodin, 1994).

Needless to say, our eating habits are also affected by the media and the context. Children are targeted by ethically questionable television commercials advertising the fast food industry (the 'happy meal') to create life-long customers (Jackson *et al.*, 2015). Another source of worry is the excessive display of sweets and snacks in supermarkets (Horsley *et al.*, 2014), which puts pressure on parents to yield to their children's demands (O'Dougherty *et al.*, 2006). What and how much we eat further depends on the people we share the table with (Shimizu *et al.*, 2014; Maykovich, 1978) and norms expressed around eating in our company (Robinson *et al.*, 2014). Again, conformity plays an important role here.

Psychology of exercise

Physical exercise has significant health benefits. It makes us stronger, promotes cardiac health and the health of the brain (Hillman *et al.*, 2008) and there is recent evidence that it stimulates the immune system (Lancaster and Febbraio, 2015). We are motivated to exercise because of the endorphins generated in the brain that give us pleasure in the short term (Gupta and Mittal, 2015) and lead to changes in the brain that benefit cognitive functioning (Thomas *et al.*, 2012). In the long run endorphins may be addictive, which motivates us to keep our exercising going. Overall exercise tends to provides us with a prolonged sense of wellbeing and accomplishment (Penedo and Dahn, 2005). In particular **aerobic exercise** – any vigorous exercise that elevates respiration and heart rate – is considered to have such benefits. In several countries, this has led to public health recommendations promoting exercise (Fletcher *et al.*, 1996).

Reviews of aerobic exercise in rehabilitation literature after or during chronic illness demonstrated improved quality of life and wellbeing (Mishra *et al.*, 2012; Bergenthal *et al.*, 2014) and cardiac health after heart failure (Heran *et al.*, 2011; Anderson *et al.*, 2016). A recent systematic review also demonstrated the health benefits of active travel, such as walking and cycling to work or school, which would not normally be seen as exercise (Saunders *et al.*, 2013). One of the problems with this type of research is selection bias: the participants have chosen to be in the exercise or activity group, which may make them different in more than one way from those in non-active control groups. For many people exercise has been built up over the years, is part of their life-style, weekly timetable, choice of friends (even partners) and social support system. Someone who has never exercised may not have these support structures in place and will therefore find it more difficult to get started and keep it going. Research shows that social support of others engaging in the same exercise is often crucial (Brown *et al.*, 2014), even if these were 'virtual' partners (Irwin *et al.*, 2012). Self-efficacy (am I good at this?) is also important (Garcia and King, 1991).

Longevity and healthy ageing

Longevity is sometimes equated with particularly healthy lifestyles, at other times with particular natural circumstances, or with genetics. Longitudinal research covering ten years (Belloc, 1973; Belloc and Breslow, 1972; Breslow and Enstrom, 1980) with almost 7,000 Californians succeeded in establishing significant longevity benefits for seven health practices:

- never smoking cigarettes;
- regular physical activity;
- moderate or no use of alcohol;
- 7–8 hours' sleep per night;
- maintaining healthy weight;
- eating breakfast;
- not eating between meals.

Many people conceive of such findings as prescriptive and resist rather than follow them. This is a common response when we feel the freedom to make our own decisions is under threat (Brehm and Brehm, 2013). The filmmaker Woody Allen famously said, 'You can live to be a hundred if you give up all the things that make you want to live to be a hundred'. Indeed, research on centenarians in Georgia shows that a virtuous lifestyle (no alcohol and nicotine, diet low in fat and meat, low stress, and continued vigorous work into old age) contributed to their longevity (Martin *et al.*, 2006). These are more or less the same factors that are associated with healthy ageing. A specific interest today is in how **brain health** can be maintained. Current evidence highlights the positive impact of aerobic exercise and being cognitively and physically active. The more sophisticated brain infrastructure resulting from life-long learning is considered a major protective factor against dementia (Hannigan *et al.*, 2015; Barnes and Yaffe, 2011).

Activity 8.4 *Reflection*

Think about a health risk behaviour that you engage in. Write down the details. If you don't have a bad habit pick one that you have seen in someone else (which is often easier, isn't it?). Analyse the behaviour in terms of its impact and stability. After reading the next section return to it and consider how your thinking has been affected.

Some thoughts are provided at the end of the chapter.

Health cognitions and behaviours

What we do to be healthy depends on how we think about health and, particularly, our own health. This is what you need to consider.

Think rationally

As we've discussed in Chapter 6, we vacillate between sophisticated (Rational Wonder) and simplistic thinking (Cognitive Miser). This also applies to how we think about health. We analyse but also ignore information. As we've seen in the section on psychology of nutrition, we are prone to be motivated by potentially unhealthy urges and it is essential to control these.

Think in positive ways

We've also discussed this in Chapter 6. Research evidence has demonstrated consistently how positive expectations make positive outcomes, including health outcomes, more likely (Carver *et al.*, 2010).

Attribute the causes of success within yourself

Attribution theory addresses how we see the causes of events in our lives. Sometimes we emphasise external causes (something in the environment), sometimes we highlight internal ones (a quality within you). We also discriminate between stable causes (it is always this way) and unstable causes (it was a fluke). People show preferences in their use of these attributional styles (Heider, 1944). For successful health behaviours we see an interesting pattern. If you ask your patients who are on a diet why they think they will succeed, these are the sort of responses you might receive, sorted by attributional style (Table 8.2).

Table 8.2: Attribution of success organised by attributional style – why do you think you will succeed with the diet you are on?

	Internal	**External**
Stable	Because I am stronger than my urges.	Because I have great support from my partner.
Unstable	Because today I have very little hunger.	Because I just read an inspirational brochure.

Internal-stable attributions are a sign of strength and predict a sustained effort (Weiner, 1988). Thus it is useful to explain your successes within yourself. You would be worried for the people who would mention any of the three other types of reasons.

We see an opposite tendency in the attribution of failure. Let us say you are trying to find out why several patients with a heart condition are still smoking. Here are some of the answers you might get (Table 8.3).

Table 8.3: Attribution of failure organised by attributional style – why are you still smoking even though you know it is bad for you?

	Internal	**External**
Stable	Because I am addicted.	Everybody in my family smokes.
Unstable	Because today I have a strong urge.	I still have a pack I don't want to throw away.

If you think along the lines of the empirical evidence, you'd say that the internal-stable attribution is most resistant to change (Weiner, 1988). It is an important message for the nurse to look at ways to change the patient's thinking, before expecting behavioural change.

If health worries disrupt your peace of mind, don't deny or resist it, take action to restore it

It is very common to deny or resist new information about behaviours we've engaged in for a long time when this information is inconsistent with what we believed thus far. It is not unlikely that we will hang on to old beliefs because we don't like to think of ourselves as being wrong or stupid for having believed incorrect information (Aronson, 1969). This is an important problem in the adoption of new health principles, not just in patients, but also in nurses, doctors and health-care institutions. New information that makes us feel bad about ourselves tends to meet with resistance (Steele, 1988). This resistance can be so powerful that we may stick our heads in the sand rather than accept that we have (stupidly) engaged in unhealthy behaviours for a long time. When we addressed cognitive dissonance theory (Festinger, 1957; Cooper, 2007) we emphasised that denial, resistance or finding justifications may reduce dissonance discomfort. However, in the long term, actions that reduce dissonance will be more effective in restoring peace of mind. Someone who wants to stop smoking but does not do so yet will continuously be reminded of the health risks. Excuses, distractions and efforts to deny or resist it will only provide temporary solace. In contrast, the cessation itself may put an end to all this. It is the same for all major improvements in health behaviour. The peace of mind that comes with thinking that you are doing the right thing is an important reward. Nurses can help with this process by accentuating the gains and helping overcome defensive responses.

Stepwise change allows our thinking to catch up with our actions and support them

Once people have actively engaged in health behaviours they did not fully believe in at first, it is likely that we will see them adjust their thinking to be consistent with their new status as non-smoker or weight-watcher. This often works best as a stepwise process in which change is contemplated, prepared for, followed by action, and hopefully maintained (Prochaska and DiClemente, 1986). Prochaska and DiClemente called this the '**stages of change model**'. While both the stages of change model and cognitive dissonance theory would suggest a natural tendency to make our beliefs and attitudes consistent with our behaviours, the pacing of this process is essential. When paced well, realistic expectations and actions will combine in likely success. However, many sudden initiatives unsupported by cognition have been abandoned when obstacles were encountered that had not been accounted for.

To round off, it is evident that understanding the mechanisms outlined here – rationality, optimism, internal attribution of success, cognitive consistency through action, paced change – is of particular importance for nurses because they provide indications for how to handle efforts to support health behaviours in patients (and themselves).

Case study: Paradoxical care

Mr Peter Jackson (71) has undergone an operation necessitated by years of drinking hard liquor. It is evident that he will have to make drastic changes to his lifestyle. He is surprisingly upbeat after the operation and quotes Oscar Wilde: 'I can resist anything except temptation.' When the nurse is taken aback by this and reminds him that surely his drinking days are over, he laughs. The next day you overhear his wife Marjory (62) discussing his funeral with him. You are puzzled by this and ask her about it. 'Well', she says, 'he will resist whatever you suggest to him. He won't stop drinking if you tell him he must. Perhaps he won't want to die, if I suggest he should.' Can you identify which cognitive aspects may play a role in this peculiar situation? How can the nurse assist Marjory?

An outline response is provided at the end of the chapter.

Stress and health

Our health is dependent on how effective we are in satisfying our needs, how well we respond to the pressures of life, how well we adjust and adapt, and how we manage the risks we encounter. Much of this is embodied in how well we cope with stress. We tend to define stress as a mental and physical condition that results from pressure or demands that are straining or exceeding an individual's capacity or perceived capacity to adapt. With the term 'pressure' we indicate the urgency of demands or expectations and the term 'stressor' can mean all conditions or events that bring about a 'stress response'.

The **stress response** is, in essence, a sympathetic nervous system response (fight–flight) which enhances our ability to respond fast and with force to emerging pressure. It is like shifting gears and highly adaptive in many circumstances, such as when we have to escape from danger. However, it can also be a problem because our system does not discriminate well between physical emergencies and situations in which we are under high pressure but should stay calm to perform well. Furthermore, long-term stress may lead to health problems. We will introduce several theories that will help you gain a better understanding of how stress affects us, accumulating in an integral model.

Case study: Models of stress (1) (to be continued)

Maryam is a community mental health nurse who visits Joyce, a senior ICU nurse who is suffering from stress and is on sick leave. Maryam is well versed in stress theory and asks her several questions that connect with models of stress.

1. How long has this been going on? Are you exhausted?
2. Are the demands in your life too high?
3. Have events accumulated in giving you stress?
4. How resilient are you normally when under pressure?
5. When you encounter pressure do you see this as a challenge you can cope with or not?

We'll come back to this case study throughout this section.

How long has this been going on? Are you exhausted? (General Adaptation Syndrome (GAS))

Stress was researched extensively in the 1950s by Hans Selye, who identified a dual physiological response to pressure via the pituitary and the hypothalamus which activates the sympathetic nervous system and the adrenal gland. Selye's (1956) massive research made use of rats that were exposed to short-term and long-term stressors. Selye looked at changes in the rats' behaviour, brain and endocrine systems and came to the conclusion that three stages (see Figure 8.1) could be identified when stressors do not abate. After the initial 'alarm reaction' the body enters a 'stage of resistance', during which the body makes fuel available (protein and fat) to keep up the high level of activation and produces several protective measures through the secretion of cortisol (for repair work) and the lacing of arteries with plaque to prevent breakage. During this stage the body is using its reserves. This eventually leads to 'exhaustion', at which point the body can no longer

General Adaptation Syndrome (Selye, 1956)

Alarm reaction: *Body resources are mobilized to cope with added stress (fight or flight response).*

Stage of resistance: *Body adjusts to stress but at a high physical cost; resistance to ether stressors is lowered.*

Stage of exhaustion: *Body's resources are depleted and stress hormones are reduced. This can result in loss of health and burnout.*

Figure 8.1: General adaptation syndrome (GAS)

keep up the high activation and is at risk of a breakdown, while the neglected immune system means that sickness becomes much more likely. Selye argued that the long-term response to stress is no different in humans.

Research in humans tends to support this claim. In particular, what happens when we reach the stage of exhaustion has been well-documented. Cardiovascular disease (House, 1974; Steptoe and Kivimäki, 2013), stomach ulcers (Crawford *et al.*, 1971; Melinder *et al.*, 2015), malfunctions of the immune system (Hall *et al.*, 2012), and abnormalities in the brain (Frodl and O'Keane, 2013) have been associated with long-term stress. Maslach and Leiter and colleagues have documented the way in which the stage of exhaustion presents itself and introduced the term '**burnout**' (Maslach *et al.*, 2001). They highlight not only the physical side but also the resulting mental exhaustion, loss of motivation, depression and a sense of hopelessness (Schaufeli *et al.*, 2009). Some of their research is particularly relevant here because it was done with nurses (Leiter and Maslach, 2009; Maslach, 2003).

Case study: Models of stress (2) General Adaptation Syndrome (Selye, 1956) (to be continued)

Maryam's questions 'How long has this been going on? Do you feel exhausted?' make sense to Joyce. She says that she has been under excessive pressure for the last year and that indeed she does feel exhausted and has lost the motivation for her work as a nurse. She has also been struggling with her physical health, with several infections in a row further depleting her energy. Maryam notes that both the duration, the exhaustion and the frequent illness fit with the pattern outlined by the GAS model. If Joyce is suffering from burnout (Maslach) a significant period of recovery may be needed.

Are the demands in your life too high? (Cannon's homeostatic model of stress)

Cannon's stress theory (Dror, 2014; Cannon, 1935) emphasises the balance between demands to the system and resources to respond effectively to them. The model suggests that the extent to which we experience stress is the result of the balance between the demands made on us

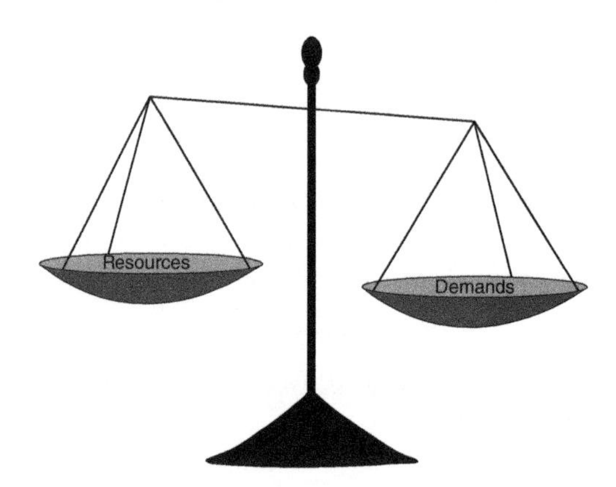

Figure 8.2: Stress and balance model (after Cannon, 1935)

and our resources (see Figure 8.2). High stress is the result of the demands exceeding resources. Not restoring the balance may have consequences for one's health, but Cannon has not really elaborated on this aspect. Nonetheless, there is evidence to suggest that actual or threatened loss of resources plays a pivotal role in the occurrence of burnout (Hobfoll and Freedy, 1993).

Case study: Models of stress (3) Cannon's homeostatic model of stress (to be continued)

Maryam's question 'Are the demands in your life too high?' makes Joyce think. She says that reduced staffing strained her. She also felt that she needed more training to lead her team. She recollects that the first time she got sick and returned to work while not fully better, she started feeling that she was not fully up to the job. Maryam suggested that Joyce list her resources and strengths and compare them with the demands. They concluded that restoring her resources of physical health and motivation needed to be prioritised. Unexpectedly, her almost two-hour commute to work appeared on the list of demands. Would Joyce be able to bring work and home closer together?

Have events accumulated in giving you stress? (Holmes and Rahe's Social Readjustment Approach)

Other approaches emphasise how stress may be the result of the accumulated need to adjust or adapt. Holmes and Rahe (1967) developed a stress measure based on this principle, emphasising common events in people's lives that require change and adjustment. The test includes a large number of life events that require the need for different degrees of adaptation, such as divorce (high degree), moving house or changing work (medium degree), and vacations or Christmas (low degree). The events are not necessarily negative but included because of the degree of adaptation required. The limitation of the model is that it assigns the same value to a certain event for everyone, while in reality events might be experienced differently and impact individuals in various ways.

Case study: Models of stress (4) Holmes and Rahe's Social Readjustment Approach (to be continued)

When Joyce is asked 'Have events accumulated in giving you stress?' she tells Maryam she is still grieving over the death of her mother six months ago and the simultaneous break-up with her partner of seven years. On the positive side, she says she met someone new four months ago but, in her present condition, she feels afraid to commit. Overall, she says it has been a very eventful year with lots of major changes.

How resilient are you normally when under pressure (hardiness and resilience)?

Several studies have since demonstrated that stress resistance (resilience) and coping factors provide indicators of how long-term stress unfolds into illness (Kobasa, 1982; Kobasa *et al.*, 1982). We differ genetically in how hardy and resilient we are and, therefore, how likely it is that we remain healthy even when we are under pressure for a long period of time. The genetic basis for these qualities is by no means uncontested, but there is evidence that there are significant differences in the extent to which we are able to effectively respond to adversity, pain and discomfort, which suggests that there is a temperamental and therefore genetic factor at work. Later in life resilience may express itself in the ability to adapt to ageing and 'improvise' effectively in changing circumstances (Gergen and Gergen, 2010).

Case study: Models of stress (5) hardiness and resilience (to be continued)

Maryam's question 'How resilient are you normally when under pressure?' makes Joyce smile. She says, 'When I first started in nursing nothing fazed me. I think in essence I've always been really strong. Also I normally enjoy exercising; I've climbed Mount Kilimanjaro, you know!' Maryam suggests that this is a good sign, which should help her. She says, 'If your old self is really strong, it is a matter of finding that again'.

When you encounter pressure do you see this as a challenge you can cope with or not? (transactional model of stress)

Lazarus and Folkman (1984) emphasised that whether the stress response takes place and how it unfolds depends not just on the stressor or pressure itself, but on how we 'appraise' it. They distinguish between two aspects. **Primary appraisal** takes place when we ask ourselves what the event means to us, whether it is important and, in particular, to what extent it is a threat or a positive challenge. **Secondary appraisal** is a reflection on whether we think we will be able to cope effectively. Recent evidence suggests that these aspects create a mind-set that is essential to how the stress experience unfolds and its impact on stress (Crum *et al.*, 2013). 'Positive appraisal' tends to work as a buffer in the reduction of the stress response (Nes and Segerstrom, 2006; Jobin *et al.*, 2014).

Case study: Models of stress (6) transactional model of stress (to be continued)

'The question "When you encounter pressure do you see this as a challenge you can cope with or not?" is all about your thinking', says Maryam. Joyce responds that at present everything scares her and she

continued . . .

continued . . .

does not feel confident she can cope. Maryam asks her to reflect on her last few days at work. 'If someone asked you how your day was, what would you have said?' Joyce responds: 'I found work hard today, I was constantly expecting the worst, and am not coping well with the pressure.' She continues, 'But a year ago I would have said: it was an exciting day, there were some interesting challenges. I needed to keep my wits about it to cope, but I always did'. Maryam says: 'We need to find a way to return to that way of thinking.'

An integrated model of stress and health for nurses (and patients)

As we've already indicated, long-term occupational stress and burnout is an important risk factor for nurses (Leiter and Maslach, 2009; Maslach, 2003; Maslach *et al.*, 2001). There is a lot of research in this area worth exploring. For now, we have tried to summarise the main findings on stress and health in a practical model that you can apply to yourself (and your patients). The model is organised in such a way that you can check whether the response to the pressures of life is likely to benefit or jeopardise health, an approach inspired by Myers (2004) (see Figure 8.3).

HEALTH RISK FACTORS	<>	HEALTH BENEFITS
	STRESS RESPONSE	
high intensity stress response	....	low intensity stress response
persistent	....	brief duration
	COGNITIVE/EMOTIONAL	
emphasis on threats	....	emphasis on positive challenge
ineffective coping skills	....	effective coping skills
pessimistic, easily depressed	....	optimistic, not depressed
	TEMPERAMENTAL/HEREDITARY	
low resilience	....	high resilience
type a-behaviour (hostile)	....	type b-behaviour (laid back)
	BEHAVIOURAL	
sedentary life style	....	regular aerobic exercise
smoking	....	non-smoking
dependencies	....	no dependencies
poor nutrition	....	good nutrition
poor sleep quality	....	good sleep quality
	OCCUPATIONAL	
high workload, low control	....	manageable workload, high control
high emotional impact	....	manageable emotional impact
	SOCIAL/ENVIRONMENTAL	
low social support	....	high social support
unsafe, frequent conflict	....	safe, infrequent conflict

Figure 8.3: An integrated model for the relationship between stress and health

The positive health-promoting elements are all on the right side of the model, while the risk factors are on the left. Let's apply it to nursing:

- **At Risk Nurse**: When I am under pressure I tend to feel physically nervous. In fact, this has been going on for months now. I tend to perceive many work events as threats, and have little confidence in my coping abilities. I also tend to be pessimistic or easily depressed under such circumstances. I don't feel very hardy when under pressure and I often get angry. My personal habits don't help. I don't take time to exercise. I smoke and drink too much alcohol and do not eat and sleep very well. I find the workload daunting and have difficulty with the high emotional intensity of the work. I am often lonely after a recent and acrimonious breakup with my partner and feel ill at ease in my neighbourhood.
- **Stress Resistant Nurse**: When I am under pressure, I tend to pace myself and make sure I relax every now and again. As a result, high stress is usually of a short duration. I tend to emphasise the positive challenge in most work-related stressors and trust that I am trained well enough to cope. I am mostly optimistic and not easily depressed. I feel resilient and easy going. I avoid drugs and drinking too much. I don't smoke. I enjoy exercising and tend to eat and sleep well. We have found ways to make the workload manageable and debrief after particularly emotional events. I take time for friends and family and enjoy their support. I am happy with my living arrangements and feel safe and rarely have lasting conflicts.

The strength of this model is in its application to one's own situation. By evaluating our own support and risk factors we may be able to establish where our strengths and weaknesses are and thus where we can make improvements. In addition, you might be interested in using a stress management workbook (Davis *et al.*, 2008), which provides useful exercises to reduce stress and its impact.

Activity 8.5 — *Reflection*

In sequence, apply each of the models introduced in the text to your own life, including your role as a nurse or student nurse. Write down your findings.

1. Selye's GAS model.
2. Cannon's Homeostatic model.
3. Holmes and Rahe's Social Readjustment approach.
4. Lazarus and Folkman's Transactional model.
5. Our integrated model.

Chapter summary

- The bio-psycho-social model of health care has mostly replaced the bio-medical model. Economic, political and spiritual factors should also be considered to fully understand contemporary health and health care. This development suggests a more holistic approach to nursing.

continued . . .

continued . . .

- A healthy diet, exercise behaviours and healthy ageing are determined to a large extent by behavioural factors and are therefore areas of psychological interest.
- Cognitive factors such as attribution theory and dissonance theory provide important explanations for success or failure to improve heath behaviours.
- Persistent stress is a very important health risk for patients and nurses alike.
- The ability to activate several stress models is important for nurses to consider different avenues in stress assessment and management.

Activities: brief outline answers

Activity 8.1: Critical thinking 2050 GP visit (see page 129)

Considering the rising costs of health care it is not unthinkable that health insurers would create a bonus point system whereby efforts to live in health protective ways would generate discounts. Perhaps the GP would be involved in the verification. Today GPs know more about illness than health. This is bound to change.

Activity 8.2: Critical thinking Mr Aziz (see page 132)

Medical concerns: was the operation performed successfully? How is the progress? What kind and length of rehabilitation expected? **Psychological concerns**: are there psychological causes to the heart condition? What are the psychological advantages of home over those of the rehabilitation unit? What are Mr Aziz's concerns? **Social concerns:** what is the role of the family in decision making? How prepared are they in providing the much-needed support? Are there cultural/religious factors involved? **Economic, political, religious concerns**: what are the costs of hospital visits to the family? Coming from Iraq are there political and religious concerns?

Activity 8.3: Critical thinking rich ←→ poor countries (see page 133)

Concerns in rich countries: obesity, physical fitness, diabetes type II, cancer. Concerns in poor countries: HIV-AIDS and other infectious diseases, hunger, poverty. There are many more differences.

Activity 8.4: Critical reflection on unhealthy behaviour (see page 136)

This exercise should give you plenty to ponder. It should provide insight into attributional and dissonance processes and how change processes might be instigated.

Case study: Paradoxical care (see page 138)

Resistance can be rooted in dissonance (Festinger) resulting from unhealthy behaviour or the fear of loss of freedom (Brehm). Perhaps Prochaska and Di Clemente's Stages of Change model can serve as a model to instigate a gradual change in Mr Jackson. The nurse could alert his wife to it. By the way, her paradoxical approach may not be without merit.

Case study: Models of stress (1–6) (see pages 139–142)

Each of these highlights the stress model discussed at that point in the text. Each model provides a different perspective on Joyce's situation.

Activity 8.5: Application of stress models to self (see page 144)

It is hoped that your analysis will have provided you with new insights.

Further reading

Marks, D., Murray, M., Evans, B. and Estacio, E.V. (2011) *Health psychology: theory, research and practice* (3rd Ed). London: Sage.

This text covers health psychology within a global, social and political context.

Ogden, J. (2012) *Health psychology: a textbook* (5th Ed). London, UK: McGraw Hill / Open University Press.

This core health psychology text combines a conceptual and sophisticated research focus.

Rice, P. L. (1999) *Stress and health* (3rd Ed.). New York, NY: Brooks.

While this is not the most recent book relating stress to health it is highly comprehensive and far from outdated.

Davis, M., Eshelman, E. R. and McKay, M. (2008) *The relaxation and stress reduction workbook.* Oakland, CA: New Harbinger Publications.

The strength of this book is in the exercises and practical stress management guidance.

Useful websites

http://www.apa.org/health/

The American Psychological Association is a rich resource on practical health psychology. A series of short videos *Psychologists in Integrated Health Care* demonstrate the role of psychologists in today's health care (These can also be accessed on YouTube).

https://www.youtube.com/playlist?list=PLD058C0C3FF56FBE2

Dealing with Stress – BBC Explorations/Storyteller Media. There are five parts to this series, which covers many aspects of stress in an accessible way.

http://www.bbc.co.uk/programmes/b01cywtq

High Intensity Training – *Horizon: The Truth About Exercise* (BBC Two). Michael Mosley's programmes are often challenging our thinking around psychology and health. This is no exception (short bits also on YouTube). Access only within the UK.

Chapter 9
The crisis of illness

Chapter aims

After reading this chapter you will be able to:

- understand how the crisis of illness unfolds and affects all involved: patient, family, work and community;
- apply the bio-psycho-social model to the crisis of illness;
- discuss how a crisis is experienced and affected by illness beliefs and cognitions, framing and inner conflict;
- relate the psychology of chronic illness to factors that impinge on it such as stress, support at home, pain, chronic fatigue, mental health, stigma, and grief.

In this chapter we look at the crisis of illness and its impact on patients, families and community. We consider the bio-psycho-social model and core perspectives on crisis, self-regulation and coping. We also discuss illness cognitions and beliefs, including framing and inner conflict. In the second half of the chapter we examine the psychology of chronic illness with specific sections on stress, home care, pain, chronic fatigue, mental health, stigma and grief. The activities will give you insight into the full complexity of how illness crises emerge and what nurses can do to help address them.

Case study: Bio-psycho-social aspects of the crisis of illness

Biological or medical aspects

At a routine check-up Christine, 55, is diagnosed with cancer. The prognosis is not favourable. Chemotherapy has been started and surgery has been discussed. Christine is often nauseous and finds her energy sapped. She studies her type of cancer and the impact of the treatment. She is on a diet and, when she can, she performs light exercises.

Psychological aspects

After a period of denial and sadness Christine is now firmly focussed on coping with her cancer. She is well aware of the seriousness of her condition, but would like to know what she can do herself. She worries about her family but succeeds in expressing herself in positive and hopeful terms. She has bad days, but tells herself it is pointless to cry. She is optimistic that she will make a full recovery.

Social aspects

Before her illness became apparent, Christine and her husband Paul were both working and sharing the care of their three small children. Paul has now taken leave from work to take care of the children. It is an unsettling period for them. Christine also paid almost daily visits to her elderly mother, who is

continued . . .

continued . . .

struggling without her help. There is no-one else who can step in. She has to give up her role as youth coach in a local sports club, which is struggling to find a replacement.

Economic aspects

The family's health insurance covers most of the costs of treatment, but the cost of driving and parking at the hospital adds up. Furthermore, Paul's time off from work reduces the income of the family and, in the long term, it puts his job in jeopardy. Child minding costs have also gone up.

Spiritual aspects

Christine and Paul do not go to a church and tend to keep their spiritual side more or less low key. The present situation has changed this a bit. Christine has started reading spiritual guidance literature and is interested in the spiritual side of recovery from cancer.

The crisis of illness

It is not difficult to see that the case study about Christine portrays a major crisis, in a medical sense but also in a psychological and social sense. The term 'crisis' indicates that events stretch or exceed the resources a person has to respond effectively (Caplan, 1964). Being in a crisis often means that people need help, feel frightened and have experiences and emotions that are new to them (Hopkins and Mackenzie, 2008). Let us look at three different models of crisis and illness.

Crisis theory and illness

According to Caplan (1964) there are three stages in most crises (see Figure 9.1).

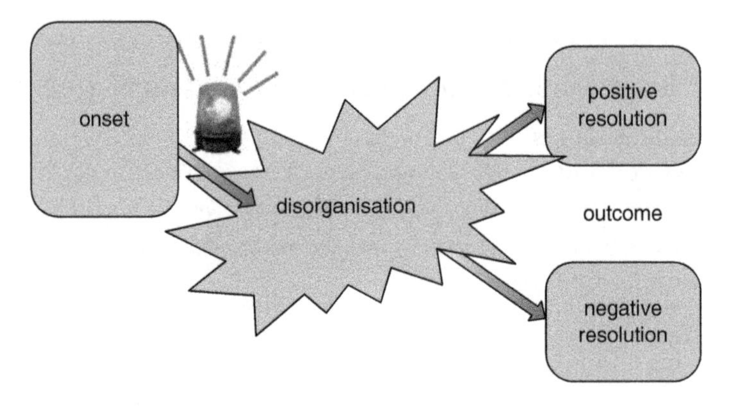

Figure 9.1: Three stages of crisis (adapted from Caplan, 1964)

During the **onset** of illness, tensions rise when it becomes clear that the problem cannot be resolved easily. A sudden onset, such as an unexpected diagnosis of cancer, will trigger a stress reaction (Selye, 1956). Stress will also dominate when long drawn out diagnostic testing is involved. If the crisis is not resolved quickly, this tends to be followed by a period of **disorganisation** during which high levels of tension and anxiety may emerge, coping mechanisms may be stretched, unpredictable responses and behaviour changes may take place and helplessness may emerge. This stage covers hospital admission, treatment or surgery and the disruption created in the lives of all involved. The third stage suggests that at some point a **resolution** will follow with positive and/or negative outcomes (Caplan, 1964). Things are rarely entirely black or white. For instance, following successful treatment or surgery there will often be lingering issues such as the need for rehabilitation or lasting diminished capacity.

This theory presupposes a homeostatic equilibrium that will be disrupted and discontinued in times of crisis. A crisis is temporary, has a sudden onset, and evokes emotional tensions that need to be resolved. The theory asserts that a crisis will disturb the normal balance between the perception of problems and the coping resources and strategies. The habitual equilibrium-restoring actions that had served the person in the past now fail.

Self-regulation and illness

Leventhal (Leventhal *et al.*, 2003) and his collaborators developed a detailed approach to understand what happens when we face the crisis of illness. They call for a 'self-regulatory model of illness', suggesting that the person actively regulates the response, including the sense-making process, emotions, and coping efforts (see Figure 9.2).

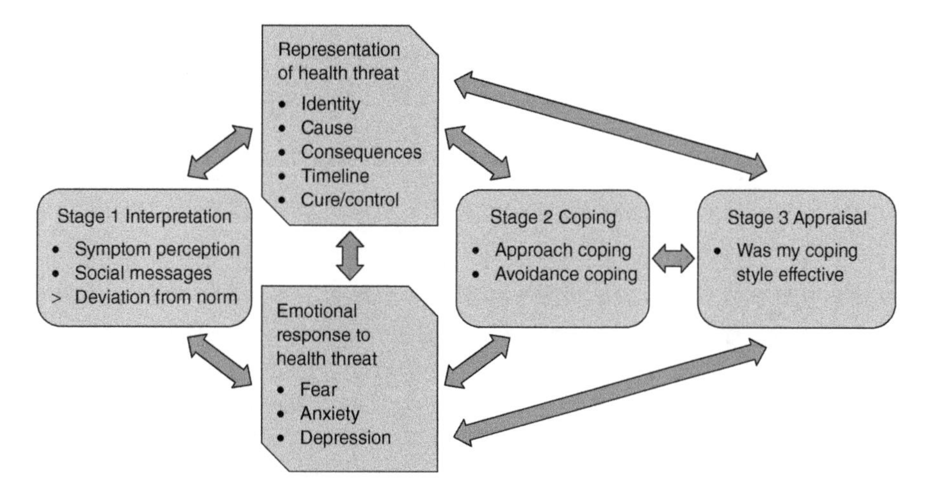

Figure 9.2: Leventhal's self-regulatory model of illness behaviour (adapted from Ogden, 2012)

Stage 1, the initial response, incorporates making sense of symptoms, diagnosis, and how it is received by others. It is likely the upheaval is accompanied by strong emotions (fear, anxiety, anger and sadness) that reflect the perceived intensity of the crisis. Leventhal considers that primary thoughts about illness will include the following aspects:

- identity (symptoms, label, diagnosis);
- perceived cause (biological, psychological, attribution processes);
- time line (acute, chronic, short-term, long term);
- consequences (pain, impeded mobility, work, sports, social contact, end of an 'exciting' life);
- curability and controllability.

This part of the model is also referred to as the common-sense model of illness representations (Leventhal *et al.*, 2003; Leventhal *et al.*, 1980; Cameron and Leventhal, 2003). A meta-analysis of the literature suggests that it is representative of how most patients reflect on their illness (Hagger and Orbell, 2003).

In **Stage 2** the emphasis is on coping with the condition. The model distinguishes between approach (addressing the illness) and avoidance (denial or trivialising). We'll come back to the coping aspect in the next section.

Stage 3 is a reflection on the effectiveness of coping approaches. Because coping is an on-going process, the appraisal may serve to sustain or refocus specific coping efforts.

Coping with the crisis of illness

Whether we think we can cope is an important aspect of how we appraise most challenging situations (Lazarus and Folkman, 1984), and therefore also illness. However, in many instances, illness emerges unexpectedly and generates unique challenges. This means that it is hard to prepare for it. Because of this, how patients cope with their illness varies considerably. An elaborate focus on coping with the crisis of illness can be seen in Moos and Schaefer's model (see Figure 9.3).

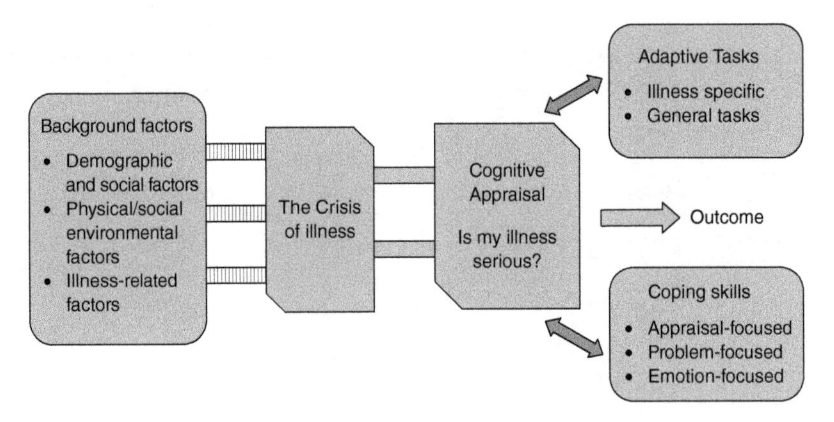

Figure 9.3: Coping with the crisis of illness. The Moos and Schaefer model (1984), adapted from Ogden (2012)

Moos and Schaefer's model highlights background factors, cognitive appraisal, adaptive tasks, and three types of coping skills (Moos and Schaefer, 1984). The background factors include demographics, physical, social and environmental aspects. The adaptive tasks include activities related to the illness such as doctor's visits, diets, medication, dealing with pain, etc. and how to rearrange one's work and social life. Furthermore, the model distinguishes between:

- appraisal-focused coping (figuring out the identity of the illness);
- problem-focused coping (addressing the illness); and
- emotion-focused coping (coming to terms with the illness mainly by expressing and regulating feelings around the illness).

In this model appraisal and problem-focused coping coincide with Leventhal's approach because both include efforts to make sense of and address the situation. And while avoidance and emotion-focused coping are different, in some cases emotional expression may be part of an evasive strategy (I feel so bad, I can't really face treatment).

Activity 9.1 **Reflection**

Discuss how Caplan's, Leventhal's and Moos and Schaefer's models apply to the Christine case study on page 147. Identify the extent of the crisis from the perspective of all people involved and consider the difference in emphasis in the three models. Following this, consider the role of the nurse. What can you do for Christine?

An outline answer is provided at the end of the chapter.

Health psychology researchers have attempted to establish which ways of coping are most effective. Their findings indicate that 'approach coping' tends to lead to better health outcomes (Kennedy *et al.*, 2010) than 'avoidant coping' (Compas *et al.*, 2012). More specifically, de Ridder *et al.* (2008) conclude from their review that, 'patients should remain as active as is reasonably possible, acknowledge and express their emotions in a way that allows them to take control of their lives, engage in self-management, and try to focus on potential positive outcomes of their illness' (de Ridder *et al.*, 2008, p. 246). Recognition of possible positive impacts of an illness include an appreciation of learning, a sense of mastery stemming from effective coping, and how it may have given new meaning to the person's life (Taylor, 1983; Taylor *et al.*, 1984). In such cases, patients seem to 'rise above' the illness. It is not uncommon for this to have a spiritual dimension. Recent evidence from a meta-analysis suggests that it may not be the coping approaches as such, but the flexibility of application that predicts effectiveness and positive psychological adjustment (Cheng *et al.*, 2014).

The strengths and limitations of the three models

The models have a broad area of application including acute and chronic illness or conditions, injury, disability and mental illness. The strength of Caplan's model is that it highlights how disorganisation and help-seeking coincide. The message for nurses is to expect strong emotions and disorganised thinking in patients. In contrast, Leventhal's model provides a clear outline of how patients may make sense of and respond to their illness, while Moos and Schaefer's contribution is in the detail of the coping process. Nurses can be instrumental in assisting patients to rise above the disorganisation (Caplan) and move towards engagement with cognitive and behavioural self-regulation (Leventhal) and active coping efforts (Moos and Schaefer). Considering the intensity of many illness crises, it is not unlikely that disorganised thinking will dominate the sense-making process suggested by Leventhal. This is the main reservation we have regarding Leventhal's model. Also, if your impression from these models is that the way in which we respond to illness takes place in neatly defined stages, you've been deceived by the separate blocks in the figures. The often chaotic reality is perhaps best understood in terms of the arrows pointing back and forth. The reality of the crisis of illness may be much more 'messy' than is suggested (see Figure 9.4). Helping the patient to create order in this process is part of your challenge as a nurse.

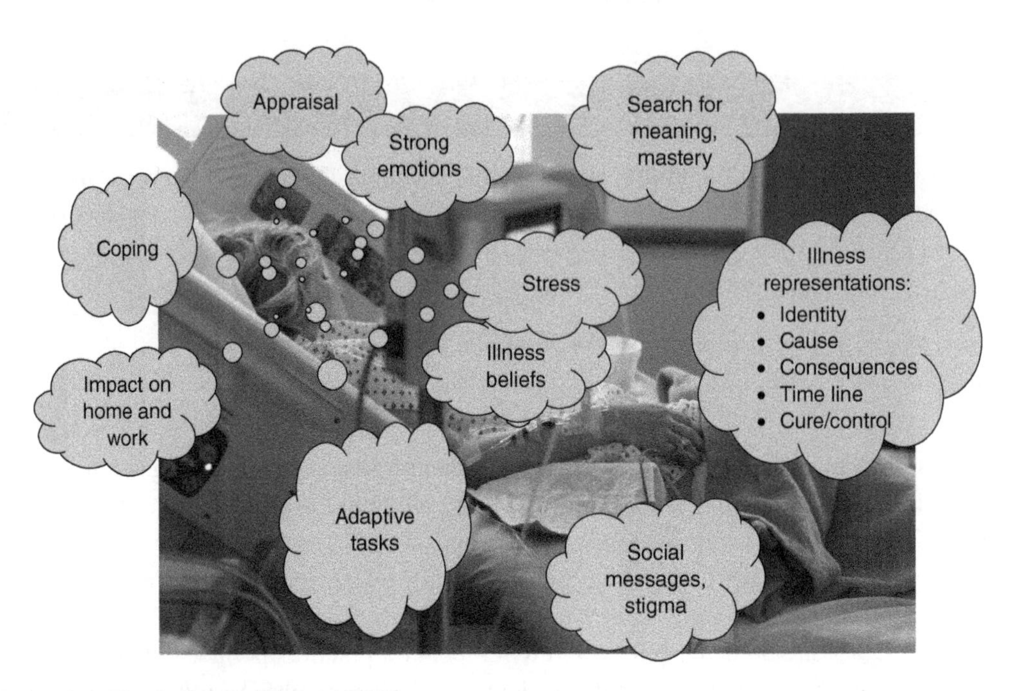

Figure 9.4: The challenge of the crisis of illness

Furthermore, the models, while including references to social aspects, put too much emphasis on the person as an independent agent and do not do enough justice to the involvement of partners, family, work and community. If we look at the social aspects of Christine's illness, it is clear that the illness generates significant problems around her. Coping is done not just by her, but also by her colleagues, her children, her husband Paul, his work, her elderly mother, and even the sports club.

Illness cognitions

It should be evident from our commentary so far that, while rational and organised thinking is preferable, all cognition, including disorganised, simplistic and biased thinking, plays an essential part in the crisis of illness. Therefore, a good understanding of processes affecting illness cognitions is important for nurses. Essentially, illness cognitions are subject to the same mechanisms as health cognitions and therefore the sections on thinking in general (Chapter 6), bias (Chapter 7) and health cognitions (Chapter 8) are also applicable here. To avoid repetition, we will focus therefore on aspects not yet addressed in detail, specifically the principles of cultural influence and framing. We will, however, return to the role of cognitive dissonance (Chapter 8) and its specific application to illness cognitions.

Case study: Culture, religion, family and illness

Aamir (53 years) has been admitted with a serious liver condition. He had been feeling pain for several months and his skin colour had become yellowish. His wife, Daneen, had urged him to go to see a doctor, but he was reluctant to do so. 'I am too busy to be sick', he would say. One day he had to be rushed to hospital by ambulance with what looked like liver failure. Following urgent intervention, his condition has stabilised, but there is damage to his liver. Aamir is angry and has trouble accepting his condition. He is particularly afraid that this will ruin his business. Thinking about the causes of his illness, he reflects back on a period in his past when he lived, as he says 'in sin', going to discotheques and drinking alcohol. Although he has left all that behind and leads a healthy life now, he says he still struggles to stay sober. He does not hesitate to proclaim that he is a devout Muslim and believes that through his prayers he ought to have avoided the disease. He also thinks that God may be punishing him for his transgressions of the past. His family tries to help him, but he finds it hard to accept advice from his wife and grown-up children who are not very religious. Consider Aamir's case when you read the next section.

Illness beliefs: cultural and individual factors

In contemporary Western society most of us believe that illness needs to be understood within the context of medical science, pharmacological interventions and surgery. We have been raised to be optimistic about medical progress and children learn from an early age that you go to the doctor or the pharmacy when you are ill. So much so that, for instance, we find it hard to accept that most colds or flu symptoms will heal of their own accord in about as much time as it would take to 'cure' it by pharmacological means. GPs will tell you that patients with a cold who do not receive a prescription often feel short-changed.

While the medical perspective has made inroads in most cultures, **traditional beliefs** and values continue to exist alongside the dominance of Western medicine. Contradictions between the two may lie dormant until health- or illness-related events trigger them. Sometimes nurses see inner conflicts within patients, or family or generational conflict that can complicate care provision. Tolerance of traditional beliefs varies in our health-care system. Overall, we are quick to point out the irrationality in deviations from the norm and are sometimes shocked when cultural or religious beliefs contravene medical protocol, vaccinations or potentially life-saving medical treatment. Interestingly, when values emphasise family ties and decision making, person-centred care can also be a matter of contention.

Having said this, it is important to realise that traditional beliefs may have an important function, especially when health care is primitive and illnesses are hard to avoid or hard to treat. Does it do any good to know that malaria is caused by mosquitoes when they are everywhere and there is no local cure? Not really, therefore people can be forgiven for preferring to believe that malaria is caused by witchcraft or adultery as they do in some parts of Malawi (Launiala and Honkasalo, 2010). Parallels can be drawn to well-known problems in industrialised countries. Does it help a family to know that asthma might be caused by pollution if they can't move to an area with cleaner air? Does it help to know that a chronic condition may be work-related if changing profession is not an option? In such cases, it may not be traditional beliefs that come to the fore, but we may use any plausible alternative explanation. We have to realise that, just as with health beliefs, the complexity and multiplicity of the information we receive from experts and the media may create confusion. Consequently, many people tend to believe what they choose to believe. We must also remember that we are often subject to confirmation bias (Nickerson, 1998). We seek support for what we believe and ignore contrary information and evidence. This tendency to simplify also occurs when patients entertain vague and 'woolly' notions of their illness, even if they have been given very precise information.

Seeking help and framing

Illness cognitions play a core role in the decision to seek medical attention for an ailment. Whether you go to the doctor depends on how the symptoms are framed. 'Framing' is the activation of a specific cognitive perspective towards a situation. In the example (see Figure 9.5) we see how framing the symptoms of a cold as a medical issue or not can have a significant effect on the actions that are taken.

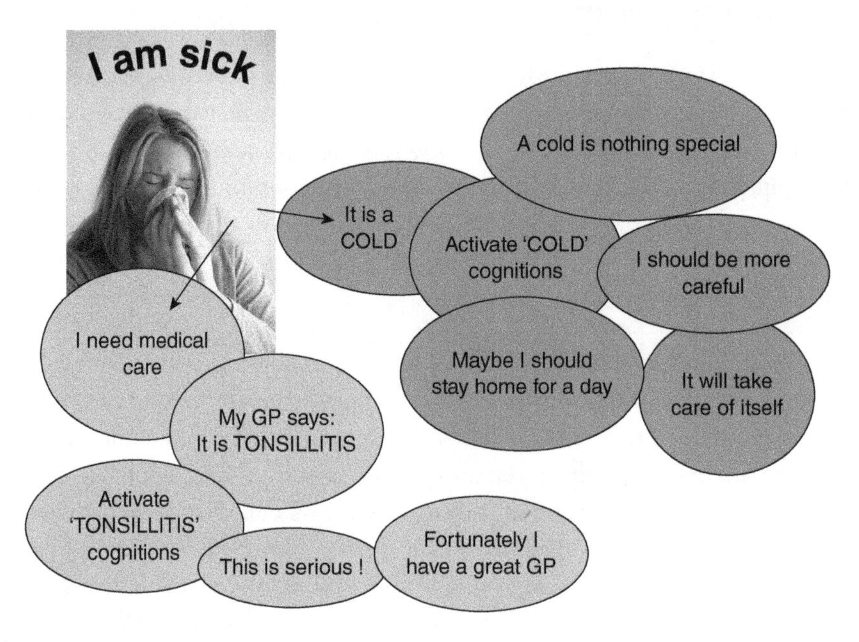

Figure 9.5: Framing of illness

In this case, it does not matter too much because regardless of the framing, the prognosis for recovery is good. In other cases active help-seeking tendencies may be beneficial because they could ensure prevention or early treatment of illnesses that are hard to battle in an advanced stage. Men tend to be more at risk of mistakenly framing symptoms as innocuous (Ogden, 2012).

Inner conflict in patients

The sense of crisis around illness is intensified when patients see themselves as responsible for their condition. If you have yourself to blame this will add to the sense of crisis. We introduced the principle of cognitive dissonance already in Chapter 5 (and 6) and explained how internal inconsistency is a source of discomfort. Being in the hospital for something you could have avoided is inconsistent with the perception we have of ourselves as smart, right, good, etc. (Aronson, 2004). This discomfort can become the source of great suffering (such as intense embarrassment, guilt, shame, regret and remorse).

Other common internal conflicts occur around decision making, such as when to visit a doctor and what kind of treatments to choose from (if there is a choice to be made). The core of these conflicts can be described as the dilemma between approach and avoidance tendencies (Lewin, 1935). For instance, going to the doctor for a health check may involve a weighing of the advantages of the reassurance of one's good health (approach) versus the rigmarole of having to go to the hospital and having to anxiously await the results (avoidance). This is called an approach–avoidance conflict (Miller, 1951). It can be a real dilemma and it is very common for people to dither, waver and spend a lot of time worrying and ruminating about what to do. There are also situations in which there is internal conflict about two positive alternatives (approach–approach conflict). The choice between different methods of pain relief during childbirth is a good example of this. Another one is the choice between two different doctors who both have excellent reputations. There are also avoidance–avoidance conflicts. For instance, in end-of-life decision making the choice between prolonged pain or death can be an intense source of internal conflict for patient and family. These possible sources of intense inner turmoil in patients require understanding and attention from those providing care. Often effective communication and information provision can help sort out an inner conflict. However, sometimes it is a matter of highly individual concern, in which the nurse can only assist by empathising and listening.

Activity 9.2 — ***Reflection***

Can you relate the Aamir case study on page 153 to the content of this chapter so far? Consider (a) bio-psycho-social aspects; (b) the extent of his crisis; (c) which cultural aspects play a role; (d) what kind of conflicts he might feel; and (e) how you might support him.

An outline answer is provided at the end of the chapter.

Psychology of chronic illness

The crisis of illness is most strongly felt in chronic illness (Frank, 2013). In fact, there is often a succession of crises, starting with the first diagnosis, followed by loss of capacity and/or hospitalisation, surgery or invasive treatment, having to learn to live with a chronic illness, and the threat of death. Depending on how fast each crisis unfolds it may be experienced as one big crisis or a succession of crises. Because the pathway of a chronic illness is at best only partly predictable, the patient's and family's coping skills may constantly be challenged. This is stressful. Generally, whatever supports the patients in reducing pressure and stress while restoring a sense of control is likely to positively affect not only quality of life but also in many cases the illness prognosis and treatment outcomes (Ogden, 2012).

Chronic illness and stress

As we've seen in the previous chapter, prolonged stress disrupts health, including the immune system, and may be part of how some illnesses start. Stress also has the capacity to exacerbate many illnesses including cancer (Powell *et al.*, 2013; Sklar and Anisman, 1981), cardiovascular disease (Steptoe and Kivimäki, 2013) and immune deficiency disorders such as HIV-AIDS (Weinstein and Li, 2015). This is particularly problematic because how do patients avoid stress when the illness itself is an important stressor? In particular, stress before surgery needs to be taken seriously. There is evidence that stress related to cancer surgery can impact the immune system and therefore promote metastasis of the cancer (Neeman and Ben-Eliyahu, 2013). Yes, you are reading it correctly; the stress of an operation to remove a tumour can increase the chances of it spreading. It stands to reason that stress management for patients should be high on the list of priorities of hospital treatment and preparation for surgery. It is an important problem that the sometimes chaotic environment in hospitals may add to the patients' stress, making them more vulnerable in an environment where the risk of exposure to hospital-based infections is high. This is an argument for sending patients home whenever it is possible.

Support at home

Support at home is essential for recovery. Typically, education and other interventions involving partners or family that include increasing the patient's active control or self-efficacy are likely to aid recovery most (Smith *et al.*, 2009; Jones and Riazi, 2011). In particular, where rehabilitation requires support at home, it is essential that this aspect is well planned and discussed with partners, family or community supports. For instance, exercise needs to be planned and practised before discharge and facilitated at home to ensure effective rehabilitation after stroke or cardiovascular disease (Anderson *et al.*, 2016; Kwakkel *et al.*, 2004).

However, when a patient comes home, the crisis of dealing with the remaining disability and recovery also comes home. The upshot from the literature is that a supportive home environment is far from a given, not least because the crisis has a destabilising influence and often impacts the mood and mental health of both the patient (Hackett *et al.*, 2005; Robinson and Jorge, 2015) and family members (Han and Haley, 1999). The patients may have become overly dependent on the hospital environment and may have acquired 'learned helplessness' (Camacho *et al.*, 2013) which may stunt recovery. On the other hand, chaos or lack of support at home may also jeopardise recovery. In the case of long-term care at home, a community health team will most likely emphasise assisting both patient and family members who provide care.

Activity 9.3 — *Decision making*

Multiple Sclerosis home care

You are visiting Pat (44) and Linda (39) at their home. Linda is suffering from Multiple Sclerosis (MS). She was diagnosed five years ago. It is now at the stage where she needs increasing levels of care from Pat. You are discussing the need for several supports in the

continued . . .

continued . . .

house with them, including a wheelchair, but also whether or not the current situation is sustainable.

To discuss the situation fully you need to:

a) identify the common course of MS (look up online and in the literature) and the bio-psycho-social aspects involved;
b) map out the kind of supports needed over time and the implications for the couple;
c) identify the different psychological implications for Pat and Linda.

An outline answer is provided at the end of the chapter.

Pain and chronic pain

Pain is an integral part of many illnesses and injuries. Moreover, pain, and especially chronic pain, has serious repercussions for a patient's quality of life. Pain is at the core of how the crisis of illness is experienced. It is just about half a century ago that the **Gate Control Theory of Pain** (Melzack and Wall, 1967) was introduced, which altered the core idea that pain could only be reduced by biological means. While this met with resistance at the time (Katz and Rosenbloom, 2015) it is now a core aspect of pain theory. Pain signals are transmitted to the brain by neurons that pass through what is metaphorically called a neural 'gate' at the top of the spine. This gate can be opened, part-opened or closed, not at will but under the influence of input from other neurons with a 'handle' on the gate. These neurons come from the body and from the brain and, as a result, other physical sensations (from the body) and mental triggers (from the brain) can affect the extent to which the pain gate is open or closed. Typically, rubbing around the area that the pain emanates from can close the gate somewhat and therefore reduce pain, but intense emotions or attention focused elsewhere can also do this.

This principle means that psychological aspects have the potential to affect the pain experience. Indeed, research has shown that pain can be reduced through relaxation, physical exercises, biofeedback, hypnosis and cognitive methods such as attention diversion, use of benign or pleasant imagery, and questioning the source of the pain (Ogden, 2012).

Research summary: Psychotherapy for chronic pain

The latest systematic review of the impact of cognitive behaviour therapy (CBT) suggests that it is only marginally effective in pain reduction (Williams *et al.*, 2012). However, a review of acceptance and mindfulness training (Veehof *et al.*, 2016) has been shown to help patients with chronic pain. A study comparing the two with an arthritis education programme in the treatment of arthritic knee pain, suggested that mindfulness and education were more effective than CBT in reducing pain and its related stress (Urquhart *et al.*, 2015). Treatment of

(Continued)

(Continued)

headaches using a variety of psychological therapies was shown to be effective in multiple systematic reviews (Huguet *et al.*, 2014). In contrast, a recent systematic review of pain interventions for neuropathic pain (pain originating from damage to sensory areas in the brain) did not suggest that psychological therapies were effective (Eccleston *et al.*, 2015). Evidently, psychology is not the answer to all types of pain, although research on headaches in particular looks promising. For nurses it may be of particular interest to build up their knowledge in this area in order to discriminate when and when not to use psychological efforts to reduce pain.

Chronic fatigue

Feeling tired all the time is a highly debilitating condition. Normally fatigue, like pain, is an adaptive signal. It tells us that we should rest. Fatigue becomes a problem when it is chronic. It is an often underestimated aspect that may add considerably to the crisis experienced by patients and their environment. Findings from a British study of psychiatric morbidity in the general population (n=8580) aged 16–74 led to the conclusion that 15 per cent of the population have classified themselves as chronically tired for a period of six months or more at some point in their lives. Chronic fatigue was significantly correlated with depressive symptoms, anxiety and sleep complaints but also with physical illness. It was more common in midlife, in women, and in the less skilled and less highly educated population (Watanabe *et al.*, 2008).

Often fatigue is a side effect of an illness, such as compromised cardiac function, or the result of medication, or chemo or radiation treatment such as is used to address cancer (Donovan *et al.*, 2013). Inflammation or alterations in the brain after stroke can also lead to fatigue (Ponchel *et al.*, 2015). Sometimes chronic fatigue is one of the main symptoms as, for instance, in multiple sclerosis (MS). In other cases, such as chronic fatigue syndrome (CFS) or myalgic encephalomyelitis (ME), fatigue is the essence. Before these syndromes were formally diagnosed people suffering from them were accused of laziness or wrongly diagnosed as depressed. While in hospital, fatigue is often considered a natural result of the circumstances, medication, disrupted sleep and activities, and surgery. Its persistence tends to become mostly a problem once the patient has been discharged. Public health nurses are therefore more likely to encounter it as a problem. It makes sense to promote cognitive efforts to reduce the mental load of tiredness. If you can't change the tiredness directly, perhaps less negative ways of thinking about it may help. However, we have to take into account that many patients would be greatly insulted if they were advised that the tiredness 'is all in their heads'.

Research summary: Treatment of chronic fatigue

Reduction of chronic fatigue is not straightforward. There are medical attempts to address it, with limited success. A systematic review indicates that there is some evidence that yoga helped women reducing fatigue during recovery from breast cancer (Sadja and Mills, 2013).

Nutritional adjustments may make a difference (Omlin *et al.*, 2013) and cognitive behavioural therapy (CBT) may also help (McCrone *et al.*, 2012). Although people with chronic fatigue are disinclined to try it out, exercise, when done in a measured way such as through graded exercise (GET), has shown effectiveness (Castell *et al.*, 2011). The gradual aspect may be essential because of the risk that exercise exacerbates tiredness or leads to unusually long recovery times (Staud *et al.*, 2015). This is because fatigue pathways in the brain and endocrine system (attenuated cortisol levels) could become sensitised. These findings call for caution. Nurses should follow the progress in this area of research.

Mental health in a health crisis

Mental health is put under pressure by lying in bed, undergoing surgery, receiving several types of medication, disability, pain, fatigue and experiencing the unravelling of the life that one has built up. No surprises there. Also, if you normally remain in balance by going for a walk, exercising, playing a game or a musical instrument, working in the garden, doing some DIY activities, or going out with friends, you will find that if these avenues of mood and anxiety regulation are not accessible, you may have difficulty remaining on an even keel. In short, it is hard to maintain mental health when suffering from a chronic illness. Less well known are the mental health side effects of inflammation (Patel, 2013) and the risk of a post-traumatic response after an operation (Bienvenu *et al.*, 2013; Davydow *et al.*, 2013; Kok *et al.*, 2015). Such impacts have been documented to require extensive psychotherapy.

At a more mundane level much can be done to keep spirits high and address the fears of patients. **Optimism** is contagious and good nurses and doctors have often become experts at spreading it. Furthermore, providing facilities for distraction, entertainment, education and social support are particularly important. Where possible, exercise programmes should be promoted as these have consistently been shown to reduce depressive symptoms (Herring *et al.*, 2012) of chronic illness. Nurses can play a pivotal role in these initiatives.

Stigma

The stigma of illness is felt as aversion, disdain and unfounded antipathy. When you are on the receiving end, you tend to feel very ill at ease, excluded or, as we say, 'stigmatised'. In today's society we are often all too aware that stigmatising others is not politically correct so we try to avoid it. However, because it is part of primitive and strong inclinations that are hard to suppress, it tends to shine through or affect our behaviour in ways we are not aware of (see the section on prejudice in Chapter 7).

The term 'stigma' has a sociological origin and was first used in this sense by Goffman (1963). Health psychologists have considered it in relation to many illnesses and disabilities. Visible disfiguration, disabilities, prosthetics, etc. may lead to stigmatisation. There is also strong stigma attached to sexually transmitted diseases and mental illness (Marks *et al.*, 2011). Many of your patients are affected by this and it adds to the crisis they experience. The expectation of being excluded by family or community, discrimination or denigration may even lead to efforts to hide the illness or refuse to talk about it. Reduction of stigmatisation starts with open communication in which unconditional respect is expressed and the use of language that disconfirms the stigma.

Activity 9.4 *Communication*

Stigma and how nurses can address it.

Part 1: *Steve (22) has just come for a visit to the sexual health clinic in which you work as a nurse. He shows signs of embarrassment and does not look you in the eyes. It transpires that he recently started enjoying his sexual freedom and, following several enjoyable sexual relationships on a recent holiday in Crete, he realised that he needed to get a check-up. Not only because he partook in unprotected sexual intercourse but also because of white discharge from his penis.*

a) Discuss how you would interact with Steve to reduce the sense of stigma he evidently experiences?

Part 2: *He is diagnosed with gonorrhea but reassured that it is eminently treatable. He is advised to ensure that he lets all his partners know, which he does. At a follow-up Steve confides in you that this has become a disaster. He had started dating a girl from work, Rebecca, and telling her led to an immediate break-up followed by public recriminations on social media and being ostracised at work.*

b) Discuss the nature of the stigma Steve experiences.
c) Also, consider situations you've encountered as a nurse in which stigma was experienced. As a nurse, what can you do to address stigmatisation when you encounter it?

An outline answer is provided at the end of the chapter.

Loss and grief

The threat of loss of life is an important part of the crisis of illness. Whenever there is the threat of loss of life, all involved – the patients, partners, family, friends, colleagues, but also nurses and doctors – will go through a process of coming to terms with it. Elizabeth Kübler-Ross (Kübler-Ross, 1969) documented this process and found that it often presents itself in five stages of adjustment:

- **Denial and isolation**: denying death's reality and isolating oneself from information confirming that death will occur. 'It's a mistake; the doctors are wrong.'

- **Anger**: asking, 'Why me?' Anger may then be projected onto the living.
- **Bargaining**: the terminally ill will bargain with God or with themselves. 'If I can live longer I'll be a better person.'
- **Depression**: feelings of futility, exhaustion and deep sadness.
- **Acceptance**: if death is not sudden, it may be accepted in the end. The person is at peace, finally, with the concept of death.

She considered that we will most likely move through the five stages more or less in the order presented. It makes sense that it starts with denial. Initially, we have no cognitive concept around our own imminent death or that of someone to whom we are close. You could also say that the information about imminent death or actual death is initially dissonant with our projections of the future. Therefore, we try to reduce the dissonance by rejecting such a diagnosis. Nurses working in intensive care or palliative care will experience these responses, so it is useful to know that denial is common. The subsequent stages are a gradual pathway to acceptance but to fully accept one's death is unlikely. Many people maintain a glimmer of hope till the last moment (Clark, 2002). Like with all stage theories, it is best to consider them guiding principles. Nonetheless, Kübler-Ross's perspective has survived over 45 years and is still considered relevant, not only in understanding responses to imminent death, but also in understanding the grief of those who are left behind (Smit, 2015).

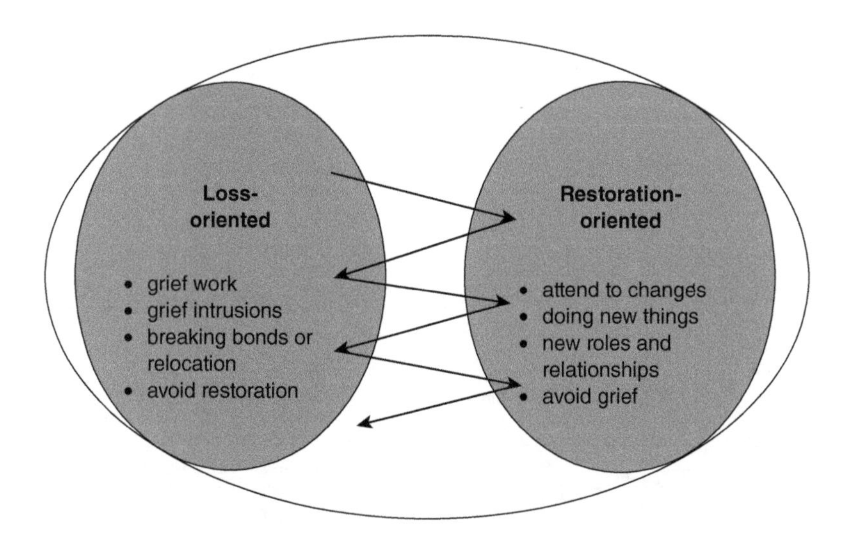

Figure 9.6: Dual process of coping with bereavement (adapted from Stroebe and Schut, 1999, p. 213)

There are several **contemporary perspectives of grief** that have moved away from the stage approach. Earlier in this chapter we have questioned overly well ordered, complex rational models of cognitive processing and are therefore pleased with the simplicity and flexibility of the dual process model of grief (Stroebe and Schut, 1999; Stroebe *et al.*, 1998). Their theory (see Figure 9.6) proposes that we vacillate between loss-oriented and restoration-oriented activities and thinking. On the one side we need to come to terms with the loss; on the other side we need to restore (if we can) our life.

Conclusion

Chronic illness can be described as a prolonged period of crisis in which stress, pressure on mental health, pain, fatigue and the possibility of loss and grief each contribute. Chronic illness is more common than ever before because people survive and have to learn to live with cancer, cardiovascular disease, HIV-AIDS and other illnesses from which they would have died in the past. Medical progress and advanced health-care systems are at the root of this. However, it is important to realise that many people have not yet adapted to this new reality. The legacy of the expectation of fatality still looms ominously over patient expectations and therefore also over how the illness is experienced. How to overcome this sense of doom is perhaps most essential to learning to live with a chronic illness. In light of this, it is not surprising – and we've already referred to this in Chapter 8 – that resilience and positive thinking are vital supportive factors (Soderstrom *et al.*, 2000; Kobasa *et al.*, 1982; Becker and Newsom, 2005).

Activity 9.5 *Reflection*

Which theme or theory presented in this chapter is emphasised in each of the following brief case studies? How should the nurse respond in these situations?

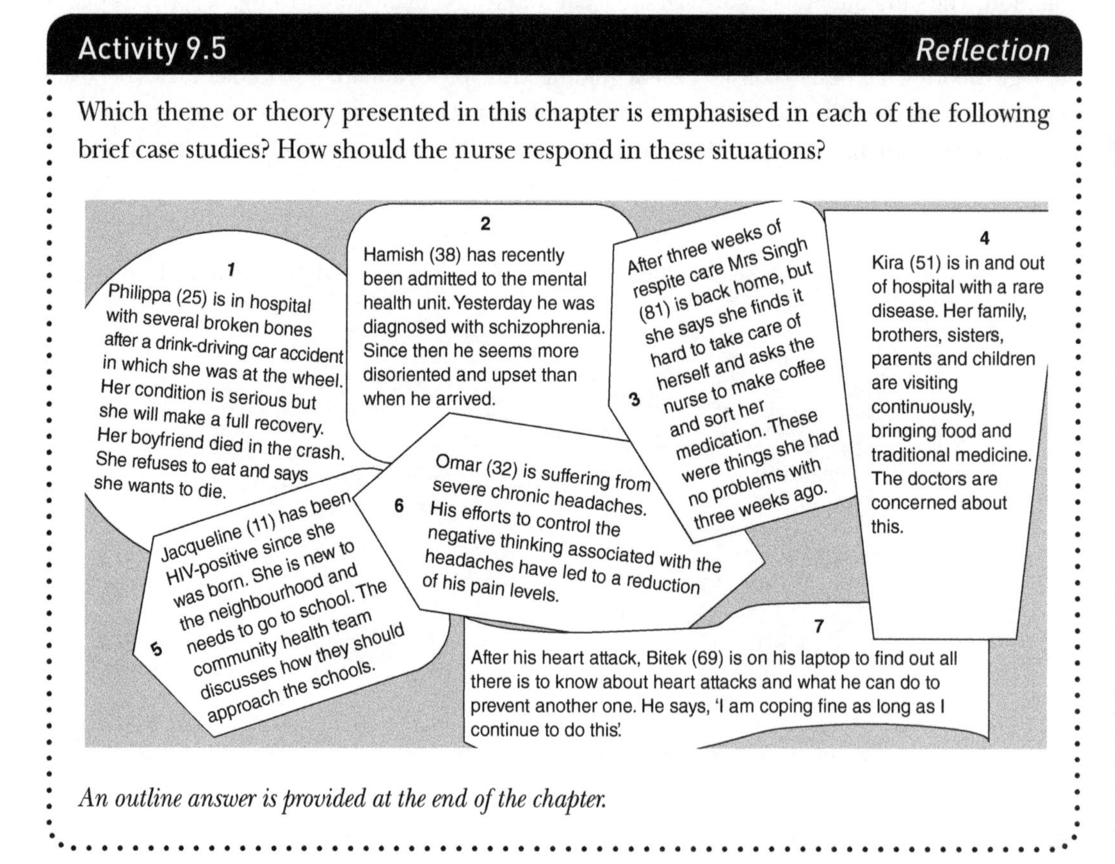

An outline answer is provided at the end of the chapter.

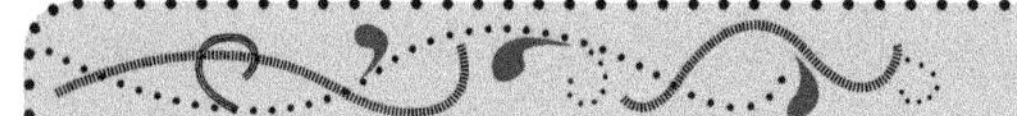

Chapter summary

- Illness needs to be understood as a crisis for the person, family and other affected parties.
- Crisis theory (Caplan) suggests that we should expect disorganised responses to illness.

continued . . .

continued . . .

- Nurses play an important role in countering this by reducing stress, supporting effective coping (Moos and Schaefer), and providing information and support that promotes self-regulation (Leventhal).
- Illness cognition is affected by the same mechanisms as health cognition.
- Beliefs rooted in our culture are not always consistent with the medical perspective on illness. This can be a challenge for patients and nurses.
- Feeling responsible for causing illness or injury through unhealthy behaviours can be an important source of inner conflict (cognitive dissonance) and mental suffering in patients.
- Stress, pain, mental health and fatigue are aspects of chronic illness that are open to psychological intervention. Nurses need to be aware of the research in these areas.
- Grief processes may take place in stages (Kübler-Ross) but there is also evidence for a dual-process of bereavement (Stroebe and Schut).
- The activities in the text will have promoted insight into the full complexity of the crisis of illness and how nurses could respond.

Activities: brief outline answers

Activity 9.1: Reflection (see page 151)

Each of the models highlights different aspects. For example: Caplan – what is the extent of the disorganisation?; Leventhal – how does Christine's self-regulation function?; Moos and Schaefer – how does she cope? At present, each model suggests that the response of Christine and her family is favourable. The nurse should keep an eye on this, provide support and information, and help them to think ahead.

Activity 9.2: Reflection (see page 155)

(a) Aamir's religion, family and work provide the backdrop of Aamir's thinking; (b) inner conflict (cognitive dissonance) regarding drinking history, not praying enough; potential generational conflict with grown-up children; (c) Aamir's suffering is not just physical but also religious, dissonance and work-related. A nurse can demonstrate empathy, understanding and provide likely and acceptable causes for his liver failure; a nurse can also rally support from the grown-up children.

Activity 9.3: Decision making: multiple sclerosis home care (see page 156)

(a) Support for Pat and Linda is a matter of helping them look ahead in terms of practical support and psychological needs; (b) because there is much information on MS, this can be used to map the future; (c) considering the grim outlook, a balance between planning for the future and a positive perspective on making the most of the present will be helpful. It is likely that Pat will need help to avoid care fatigue; Linda's coping approach needs to be monitored as continued problem-focused coping may overburden her; focus on the meaning of life and what pleasures remain is essential.

Activity 9.4: Communication: stigma (see page 160)

(a) Steve feels highly guilty (dissonant). The nurse could exacerbate it and thereby increase the experienced stigma. The nurse could also normalise his gonorrhoea and thereby open up communication channels about it, which he needs to contact whoever he has had sexual contact with; (b) sexually transmitted diseases are a source of stigma, although gonorrhoea is low on the scale; (c) regardless of your experiences, effort to communicate openly and normalise the potentially stigmatising condition will most likely have a positive impact.

Activity 9.5: Reflection (see page 162)

1) Inner conflict/dissonance; 2) disorganised stage in crisis, stage of denial, anger (Kübler-Ross); 3) learned helplessness; 4) cultural differences in illness beliefs; 5) stigma; 6) psychological approaches to pain management; 7) problem-focused coping. In each of the situations the nurse's approach will require an understanding of the perspective of the patient and support of self-regulation.

Further reading

French, D., Vedhara, K., Kaptein, A. A. and Weinman, J. (Eds.) (2010) *Health psychology* (2nd Ed.). Chichester, UK: BPS Blackwell (John Wiley and Sons).

This is another Health Psychology text to further your knowledge in this area. This one is published by the British Psychological Society (BPS).

Frank, A. W. (2013) *The wounded storyteller: body, illness, and ethics.* Chicago, IL: University of Chicago Press.

This text – and there are many others – provides the much-needed perspective of the person with long-term illness. Essential reading for nurses.

Cameron, L. D. and Leventhal, H. (2003) *The self-regulation of health and illness behaviour.* London, UK: Routledge (Taylor and Francis).

There are several texts that represent Howard Leventhal's perspective quite well. This edited text is particularly rich.

Goffman, E. (1963) *Stigma: notes on the management of spoiled identity.* Englewood Cliffs, NJ: Prentice Hall Inc.

This is a classic text on stigma that keeps appearing in new editions.

Useful websites

https://www.learner.org/resources/series138.html#

The famous *Discovering Psychology* series hosted by Prof. Philip Zimbardo. Watch nr 23: Health, Mind and Behavior.

http://www.ms-uk.org/

The MS-UK website provides a good example of online support for a particular chronic illness. Nurses can learn a lot from such websites.

http://www.breastcancer-matters.eu/

This Pfizer (pharmacological company) sponsored website presents several perspectives on breast cancer. This will help deepen your understanding of the bio-psycho-social way of looking at illness.

http://www.louisehay.com/

Louise L. Hay is the bestselling author of *You Can Heal Your Life.* This is her website. Judge for yourself!

http://www.apa.org/helpcenter/chronic-illness.aspx

The American Psychological Association (APA) has a page on coping with chronic illness.

Chapter 10
The psychology of care in practice

Chapter aims

After reading this chapter you will be able to:

- understand the role of psychology in day-to-day nursing activities;
- apply and develop principles of behavioural, cognitive, humanist and positive psychology in your care;
- identify how psychological principles benefit reflection and how this improves the quality of your work;
- discriminate between automated and unexamined practice and reflective practice.

In this final chapter we will apply psychology to the most common aspects of the care-giving role. We've already established that psychology is an essential element in health and illness, and in each of the previous nine chapters we have sought to link psychology with nursing. Now we are going to look at day-to-day nursing activities and the ways in which psychology may help increase their effectiveness. We have highlighted eight different schools of thought in psychology in Chapter 2 and demonstrated that each of them can be applied to nursing. However, four of these inform your daily care activities most: the humanistic, behavioural, cognitive approaches and positive psychology. Of the other perspectives, the psychodynamic, evolutionary and psycho-biological approach addressed in previous chapters are relevant as ways of thinking around health and illness and should be kept in mind. Social psychology has been addressed and applied in detail in Chapter 7.

Humanistic, behavioural, cognitive and positive psychology principles of care

Whenever your care efforts are focused on making a person feel better, you most likely emphasise compassion, good listening and other aspects of the humanistic approach. When you are trying to affect a patient's thinking you will be using cognitive principles, such as persuasion and providing information. When your care is focused on affecting behavioural aspects you will consider behavioural principles such as encouragement or modelling. The starting point may be different but, because feelings affect thinking and behaviour and vice versa, each approach may have an equally comprehensive impact on the person in your care (see Figure 10.1).

This interactive principle is essential to understanding how you use psychology as a nurse and how you may shift focus between these three approaches or use them in tandem. You may use empathy to directly affect a person's feelings, but those feelings may also change as a result of engaging in

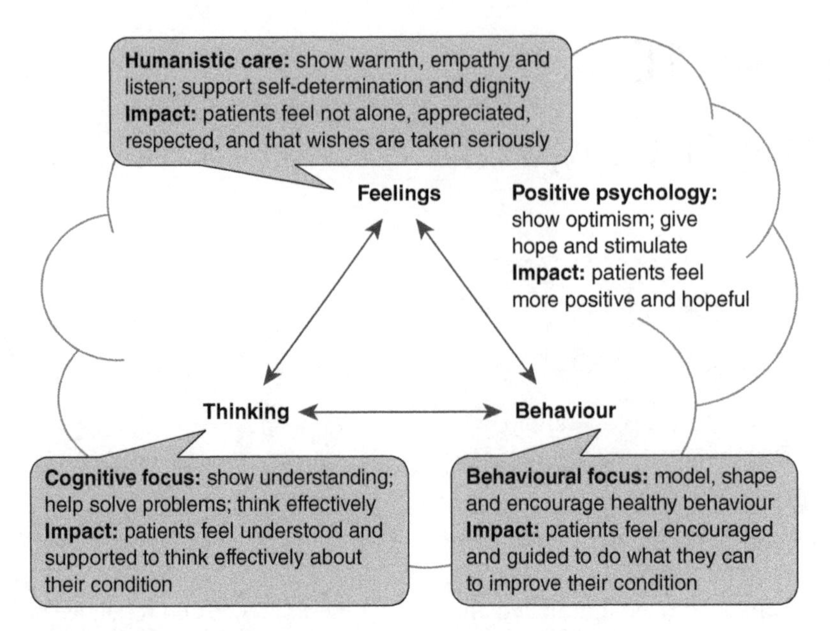

Figure 10.1: The humanistic (focus on feelings), cognitive (thinking), behavioural (behaviour) and positive psychology (overall) approach in patient care and its impact on patients

an activity or after being persuaded to think in a different way. Overall, your efforts will be more effective if they are infused with positivity and optimism, which brings in the importance of positive psychology. Positive psychology should be seen as enveloping the other three approaches.

Humanistic care: affecting patients' feelings

Humanistic principles are the basis of all core values in nursing and specifically of **person-centred care**. Humanistic principles accentuate providing emotional support (Roach, 2013). So, for instance, if you deal with a crying patient you will directly try to affect the patient's emotions that cause the crying, such as fear, sadness or anxiety. You will do your best to show empathy and listen to the patient. It is likely this support and the opportunity to express feelings will relieve anguish. The humanistic therapeutic approach is non-directive, which means that telling people what to do or what to think is not part of the approach. As we've seen in Chapter 2, the person-centred approach to nursing is rooted in Roger's work on client-centred therapy. Being effective in the use of the humanistic approach means educating and training yourself in showing empathy, listening well, being respectful, mirroring feelings, and avoiding dehumanising patients (inadvertently). There are countless ways in which we can do it right and there are many ways in which we can do it wrong (see Activity 10.1).

Activity 10.1 *Communication*

Humanistic care in practice

Discuss the difference between the **humanising** and **dehumanising** approaches presented here. Include your experience with the examples and the impact on people in your care.

continued . . .

continued . . .

Humanising	Dehumanising
Friendly greeting	Read chart before greeting
Two-way communication: also listening	One-way communication: telling them
Display empathy	Show pity
Make eye contact, smile	No eye contact
Involve patient in nurse/doctor exchanges	Talk about patients in their presence
Sitting down to talk	Exclusive emphasis on task at hand
Acknowledge pain and discomfort	Impatience with patients
Display understanding of patients	Talking down to patients
Good communication	Use of jargon
Be respectful	Rudeness/carelessness
Acknowledge uniqueness of people	Prejudice and stereotyping
Show unconditional respect	Show rejection or disdain
Give full attention	On mobile phone while giving care
Greet and acknowledge visitors	Ignoring patients' visitors

An outline answer is provided at the end of the chapter.

Operating consistently in a humanising way sounds straightforward enough but, as you can see in Activity 10.1, there are pitfalls. Avoiding these is important, but we need to do more. Because patients are vulnerable and excluded from much of family, work and community support, we will need to compensate for their loss of control, belonging and self-esteem (Bastian and Haslam, 2010). In short, nurses need to be prepared to **re-humanise**, especially when people are in long-term care.

Behavioural aspects of care: affecting patients' activities

As a nurse you are highly likely to incorporate elements of the behavioural perspective in all situations in which active engagement by the patient is required, in changing behaviour or learning new behaviours. At the core of the behavioural approach (see Chapter 2) is also the realisation that stimuli in the environment prompt emotional responses, and that such responses can become conditioned. Think of white-coat phobia, fear of blood, traumatic stress responses and other forms of conditioned anxieties and sensitivities. The behavioural approach makes use of **reinforcement** (reward or encouragement) of healthy behaviours and **discouragement** of dangerous or unhealthy actions. Overall, encouragement is more effective than discouragement because it generates positive feelings in the relationship between nurse and patient. Generally, the old adage to use the 'carrot' rather than the 'stick' (Skinner, 1938) mostly holds in health care.

Activity 10.2 *Reflection*

Behavioural care in practice.

Think of an example in which someone in your care needs to be stimulated to be active. Outline your use of encouragement, modelling and other aspects of the behavioural approach.

An outline answer is provided at the end of the chapter.

Using the same example of a crying patient, the nurse using a behavioural approach might say, 'Let's get you out of bed and take a little walk to make you feel better'. The behavioural approach is directive and may provide a firm support at times when patients are not at their best at making decisions or when they lack motivation.

Cognitive factors in care: affecting patients' thinking

Cognitive factors play an important role in how patients experience their illness. The cognitive approach to care addresses the way in which your patients think about undergoing surgery, disability, pain and the impact of the crisis on their lives.

Patients who have adopted rational and positive ways of thinking about their illness are likely to suffer less than those who are dominated by negative or irrational thoughts. Taking patient's thinking into account includes understanding cognitive strengths and limitations. This was addressed in the 'Rational Wonder versus Cognitive Miser' approach to thinking (see Chapters 2 and 6). For nurses, the cognitive perspective is explicitly included in promoting adaptive, rational, realistic, hopeful and positive ways of thinking. This starts with being interested in what patients think and how it affects them.

Activity 10.3 *Communication*

Cognitive approach in care.

Someone in your care says: 'What is the point of trying to recover? Things will never be the way they were'. Outline your efforts to assist this person to think in more positive ways.

An outline answer is provided at the end of the chapter.

Coming back to the example of the person who was crying before an operation, you might assume that it could be thoughts about the operation that precipitate the crying. You may try to dispel fear-provoking thoughts and instil hope in the patient. Nurses need to learn to identify when negative and irrational thinking or disproportionate focus on what can go wrong (catastrophising) may be affecting the patient. You may consider principles used in cognitive behavioural therapy (CBT) to further advance your expertise.

Positive psychology and combining it with humanistic, behavioural and cognitive perspectives in care

If you do it right your care efforts are infused with a positive energy and outlook. As we've already discussed, this will work as a **positive contagion**. The people in your care will be more responsive and open to you and will look forward to your presence, which provides you with a better opportunity to affect their condition. Positive psychology combines with the humanistic approach when you learn to listen and show empathy, while avoiding the trap of leaving the patient more miserable than before. The expression of life-affirming positive energy and hope will make you succeed in doing so. Positive psychology is equally essential in ensuring that the cognitive aspect of care does not remain limited to cold rationality. It is one thing to help your patients to think realistically but, without an optimistic element, this manner of thinking is unlikely to be embraced. In regard to efforts to impact behaviour, it has already been demonstrated that encouragement and reward of desirable behaviours is more effective than discouragement of undesirable responses. Thus, even in shaping behaviour, it is positive psychology that provides a vital ingredient.

In daily care you will find yourself combining these four approaches in many situations, often without thinking about it. This is fine because you don't always have time to question how you conduct your care activities. However, to develop your skills you need to become aware of how you perform them. You will then realise that you will turn to what you are learning here about humanistic, behavioural, cognitive and positive psychology. Activity 10.4 gives you an example of how it works in practice.

Activity 10.4 — *Critical thinking*

Example of combined application in care.

For each of the seven segments in the sequence, identify whether a humanistic, behavioural, cognitive or positive psychology approach is used. Segments may include more than one approach.

	What happens	Nurse reflection	Humanistic, behavioural, cognitive and/or positive aspects
1	It is morning. The nurse enters the room and opens the curtains. 'Good morning Arlene. Ah the sun is shining. Looks like a nice day.'	By expressing a positive perspective on the new day, I may affect Arlene's thinking about today in a positive way.	

continued . . .

continued . . .

What happens		Nurse reflection	Humanistic, behavioural, cognitive and/or positive aspects
2	There is little response from Arlene (the patient). The nurse turns to the patient and in a soft voice says: 'How are you doing?'	By toning down my voice, I demonstrate that I have noted that Arlene is not feeling so well. Making personal contact is best started with an open question. In my voice I try to show empathy.	
3	Arlene says, 'I am fine'. However, the tone of voice and facial expression suggest the opposite. The nurse says 'You don't sound all that great. Let me look at you.'	What Arlene says is not consistent with my other observations. Perhaps she is just trying to be polite. I better reflect my impression to the patient to demonstrate that I understand and to express my concern.	
4	'Are you in pain?' 'Are you thinking about the operation tomorrow?'	By asking direct questions about Arlene's feelings, thoughts and concerns, I may be saving time, while showing that I am aware of what she is dealing with.	
5	Arlene says: 'I am not sure.' The nurse responds by nodding patiently and waiting for additional expressions. After a moment the patient says: 'I am in pain, but I am really scared, I am so afraid that it will all go wrong.'	It is important to allow Arlene to think. My silence is an invitation to say more. I am expressing my interest in her in this way. It works because Arlene ends up expressing what is bothering her.	
6	The nurse says: 'If you want, I can go over the operation with you again in a moment.' Arlene nods affirmatively.	I could address the pain, but she has just received analgesia. Perhaps Arlene's thoughts about the operation are more important right now. I am afraid to attend to her feelings too much when my hunch is that I might be able to dispel some of her fears by discussing the detail of the operation.	

continued . . .

continued . . .

What happens		Nurse reflection	Humanistic, behavioural, cognitive and/or positive aspects
7	The nurse continues: 'In the meantime, perhaps you can walk with me if you want, while I get the documentation. Shall we talk in the meeting room? What do you think?' 'Okay', says Arlene, and starts getting out of bed. 'Give me a moment and I'll follow you.'	I want to get Arlene out of bed. This may provide distraction and perhaps reduce her pain. She may also be more alert after having been on her feet for a bit. This way the impact of our conversation on her thinking about the operation may be optimised.	

An outline answer is provided at the end of the chapter.

Psychology and day-to-day nursing duties

In this section we will address practical psychological aspects of each of the tasks in Table 10.1. We will highlight specifically how humanistic, behavioural, cognitive and positive psychology perspectives will help you to perform these activities in optimal fashion.

Table 10.1: Nursing duties
Interactions with people in your care (non-technical)
• Providing emotional support
• Communication about care planning
• Preparation for surgery and care following surgical procedures
• Rehabilitation
• Symptoms and pain management and support
• Health promotion, advice and education
Technical nursing tasks
• Diagnostics and interventions (for example, vital signs, diagnostics, wounds, infusions)
• Medication management
• Emergency responses (such as CPR)

(Continued)

Table 10.1: (continued)
Other
• Develop and update patient care plans, hand over, record keeping
• Interactions with multidisciplinary team
• Mentoring and being mentored
• Interactions with family and other visitors
• Hygiene and safety activities, non-nursing tasks
Critical reflection

Interactions with people in your care (non-technical)

Emotional support

The people in your care need emotional support. Demonstrating empathy is at the core of this: 'As caregivers, we know the importance of empathy. Trying to understand another person's perspective is critical to our profession. Increase your ability to be empathic by honing your approachability. Practice solid listening skills, use direct eye contact, and maintain an open stance' (Lachman, 2001, p. 41). It helps if you are genuinely curious and not afraid to ask questions. Don't forget that a good question to a patient is a great way of making contact and hence showing emotional support. Good listening draws on a combination of the humanistic and cognitive approach. It is very comforting to be listened to really well, a bit like taking a hot bath. Listening well requires practising several core principles and skills (see Theory summary).

Theory summary: How to calm down patients who are upset or angry

1 Listen to the story, ask for clarification, check understanding, keep your voice down, sit with the patient rather than standing over them.
2 Acknowledge the person's upset, anger or other emotion.
3 If the patient is angry at something that happened in the hospital, don't defend it until you fully understand the complaint.
4 Apologise (for the organisation) and/or explain if necessary.
5 Offer something you can do for the person.
6 At this point anger has usually dissipated and the patient will have calmed down.

Please note:

- If patients keep repeating a complaint, it means they don't feel listened to.
- Don't mistake anger for aggression. Anger is a perfectly normal response to aggravating situations.

- Keep in mind: your angry patient may be right!
- Also remember that effective listening may prevent anger from turning into aggression which is an important problem in UK hospitals (Winstanley and Whittington, 2004).

Expressing empathy and compassion starts with the realisation that you don't need to wait until you feel it. **Empathy or compassion** is something that you do! If you feel compassion but don't express it, it is useless to the patient. We would therefore say, start by expressing it and 'fake it until you make it'. Of course, to empathise with patients you need to feel a bit of what they are feeling (Gonzalez-Liencres *et al.*, 2013). It is a matter of putting yourself in their position and feeling enough of what they are experiencing to understand them. This requires awareness or 'mindfulness' (Langer and Moldoveanu, 2000). Sometimes the sheer immensity of the person's suffering can be overwhelming. At such times emotions are hard work for nurses (Gray, 2012). We call this **emotional labour** (James, 1989). The term **compassion fatigue** (Joinson, 1992) indicates how, over time, nurses may find it hard to do this and remain compassionate. Research shows that the accumulation of hopelessness in patient situations, the inability to alleviate suffering, high workload, and personal difficulties in the nurse's life may trigger compassion fatigue (Yoder, 2010). Learning to regulate your own feelings and thoughts when you are compassionate is at the core of protecting yourself and securing your long-term ability to provide compassionate care.

Communication about care planning

Considering the vulnerability of patients it is evident that the onus is on the nurse to ensure that patients understand all communication about care planning. It is important to verify comprehension and foresee possible confusion. Contemporary understanding of communication highlights that there are many ways in which misunderstandings can occur, not least because the perspective of a situation in which the communication occurs may differ radically between the communicator and the person receiving the communication (Schramm, 1971). This is very much true for nurses and patients who have profoundly different frames of reference in relation to health care, hospitals, surgery and so on.

The nurse should therefore first probe the patient to get an impression of their knowledge levels and frame of mind, mood, emotions, and cognitions related to the crisis they are most likely experiencing. The nurse might also look into which type of communication best suits the patient. Some people need to first and foremost hear the information; others need to read it or prefer a visual aid such as a diagram. Most often **multiple representations** increase the chance that information will be received in the best possible way (Ainsworth, 1999). Other relevant aspects of how to give information, and which biases to expect, have been addressed in Chapters 6 and 7. It is important to take this into account. For instance, what you say first may colour all subsequent information. Also, what is said first and last tends to be remembered better. In conclusion, it is evident that the 'cognitive mode' dominates this task for the nurse, as you will be looking at cognitive abilities, limitations, biases and preferential processing styles of your patients and yourself. At the same time you will be maintaining a humanistic perspective as you ensure that you maintain rapport with the patient during your communication.

Activity 10.5 *Communication*

A person in your care is receiving new medication. The pills are different, the dosage is different and frequency and time of taking the medication is different. It is very important to avoid confusion. Consider more than one way in which you can instruct a patient in its use.

An outline answer is provided at the end of the chapter.

Preparation for surgery

Everything that is represented in the section above is also relevant when you prepare patients for surgery. Besides, you need to take into account that many questions tend to emerge after an information session rather than during it, because the patient may be preoccupied with efforts to reduce anxiety and stress about the operation. In fact, stress reduction should be one of the main emphases of pre-op preparation. Research has shown that stress-coping techniques (Langer, *et al.*, 1975), and several other stress management approaches, including the use of soothing music (Nilsson, *et al.*, 2005; Vetter *et al.*, 2015), can facilitate post-operation recovery and reduce pain. The importance of pre-operative stress management even extends to the fact that stress can exacerbate the risks of the operation itself (Neeman and Ben-Eliyahu, 2013). The overall principle that the **stress of surgery** is problematic is far from new (Janis, 1958). Today the impression prevails that whatever nurses can do to reduce stress in patients around surgery may provide benefits. This may be through simply being with the patient and providing support by attending to feelings and listening (humanistic approach), suggesting activities that help the patient relax (behavioural) and providing assistance with coping methods that address the cognitive appraisal of the operation (cognitive). Presenting a positive and hopeful perspective (positive psychology) tends to be beneficial and even selective information-giving may sometimes protect the patient (de Vries and Timmins, 2016b).

Activity 10.6 *Critical thinking*

Under what circumstances can nurses justify selective information-giving? Debate an example and list the pros and cons and possible ethical issues.

An outline answer is provided at the end of the chapter.

Rehabilitation

Rehabilitation means recovering or relearning skills or learning new skills to compensate for loss of abilities. The behavioural approach is essential here. Rehabilitation centres specialise in this, but we would argue that it is also part of what nurses should do. Consider the following Case study.

Case study: Anna recovers from surgery

Anna (83) has had a lifesaving operation on her aorta. During the operation a tear in her aorta burst. This resulted in considerable reduction in blood flow to the brain for over ten minutes. This would have left most people severely disabled. Therefore, when Anna was recovering in the intensive care unit, hopes among nursing staff and family were tempered. One nurse, Jo, who was on duty during the week showed considerable determination in her efforts. She kept communicating with Anna, speaking to her, and seeking a response. After three days responses started to become more coordinated. Eye contact became better and there were initial efforts to speak. Jo kept looking for signs of progress in terms of motor function, understanding, speech and social contact. She said, 'Whenever I saw that Anna could do something with my help, I would focus on this aspect. So if she wanted to let me know something I would work with her to get it clear. I also tended to try out simple actions, such as eating and drinking. Once she could swallow, we step-by-step developed eating and drinking independently. First providing support and then gradually removing it as she was recovering her abilities. Every step of the way I would encourage her and coach her forward.'

Anna and Jo's story demonstrates three core principles of rehabilitation. Firstly, we need to observe and initiate the activities that the patient would need to learn to regain independence. Once able to perform a particular activity with help, we would say that the patient is in the **zone of proximal development**. Vygotsky (1978) introduced this principle as an indicator of learning potential in children, but it can also be applied to adults, especially when they are relearning skills after injury, a stroke or surgery. Secondly, we need to figure out how we can support the activity in stages and, as the person is learning, gradually remove that support so that the person becomes independent. This is called **scaffolding** (Wood *et al.*, 1976). It is essential that the scaffolding or support promotes the development, is adapted as required, and is removed gradually. Both late and premature removal of support tends to stunt independent learning. The third aspect is to ensure that the patient is motivated to engage in the process of behavioural **shaping**. Progress may be intrinsically rewarding, but often there is effort, frustration, fatigue, and sometimes pain, involved. For instance, in rehabilitation after stroke, patients may be prone to give up. It is important therefore to provide plenty of reinforcement and encouragement. As described in Chapter 4, reinforcement tends to work best when it is given immediately after the desired behaviour is performed. Nurses need to be aware of this and, furthermore, to find out what works and what does not work for an individual. In general, kind words such as 'well done' or encouragements such as 'you can do it' go a long way. But it is important to find out from patients what they like and what makes them feel good and use this. A word of warning is appropriate here because there is evidence that nurses sometimes use reinforcement in an undesirable way, in fact to discourage independence. Baltes and Skinner (1983) found that nurses unintentionally encouraged dependent behaviour and passivity in patients, particularly by discouraging leaving the bed or taking other initiatives.

In order for a rehabilitation process to work most effectively, you need to be proactive and identify progress. This applies to learning to eat, drink, walk and use the toilet independently again after an operation, learning to use crutches or other supports, physiotherapy, self-care, preparing meals, use of media, phones, computers, etc. Some of this you may normally leave to experts, such as physiotherapists, but at the initial and often crucial stage, it may very well be up to you to initiate core skills such as drinking or eating independently. Of course, whenever a learning process goes beyond practical skills but involves understanding, you will move beyond the behavioural approach outlined in the above and make use of cognitive principles. Throughout the process – we don't mind repeating it – the therapeutic relationship is rooted in the humanistic perspective and you will motivate patients using positive psychology.

Activity 10.7 *Decision making*

An older adult in your care has been given a series of yoga exercises to reduce chronic pain. The exercises include three challenges that the person cannot perform independently: standing on one leg; getting up after lying on the floor; and a forward bend with the upper body while sitting on a chair. Consider the principles of 'zone of proximal development' to address the feasibility of the exercises and 'scaffolding' to create a plan to support the exercise programme. Be imaginative!

An outline answer is provided at the end of the chapter.

Pain management and support

Most pain management is pharmacological in nature but, since Melzack introduced the **Gate Control Theory of Pain** (Melzack and Wall, 1967) it has become clear that other means of pain reduction are possible. Research has since demonstrated that relaxation, anxiety reduction, distraction, and cognitive and behavioural techniques can be used to help reduce pain (Katz and Rosenbloom, 2015). This means that, as a nurse, you should learn these techniques for use when pharmacological means are exhausted or undesirable. Because there are no known side effects, there is scope to combine different approaches until something works. Interestingly, one systematic review demonstrated that nurses' empathy was not a factor in pain reduction (Watt-Watson *et al.*, 2000). It is hard to think that the humanistic approach would not play a role in pain relief but, on the other hand, perhaps the emphasis on feelings is the opposite of what is needed.

Health promotion, advice and education

Health promotion is a matter of information-giving, educating and giving advice to promote healthy behaviour and to stop unhealthy behaviour. Theory and research on **persuasion** is most relevant to this area. In a nutshell, it suggests that you need to adapt your approach to the person you are trying to persuade, their present attitudes, levels of knowledge and motivation (Petty and Cacioppo, 1986; Upton and Thirlaway, 2010). For instance, well-informed patients will need more detailed and better-argued reasoning of pros and cons of treatment, while an anecdote or slogan might convince less well-informed patients. There is a considerable body of research specifically focused on health promotion (Brown, 2015; Raczynski and DiClemente, 2013). For the nurse the main concern is how to be persuasive when providing advice and be critically aware of relevant health promotion sources (brochures, books, videos, web-sites, support groups, etc.).

You are essentially trying to change people's behaviour through encouragement and continued support (behavioural, humanistic and positive) and through affecting their thinking (cognitive).

Activity10.8 *Communication*

Persuasion

Imagine a situation in which you need to persuade someone who is showing signs of low mood to get out of bed. Consider a hypothetical scenario and how you will go about it.

An outline answer is provided at the end of the chapter.

Technical nursing tasks

Diagnostics and interventions

It is evident that you need a behavioural, humanistic perspective as well as your cognitive and positive hat on when you are performing diagnostic tasks or interventions. Your main challenge is to learn to perform the tasks correctly and safely (behavioural), while developing an approach that maintains the humanity of the person (humanistic). The more complex the task, the more difficult it is not to treat the patient as an object. It may help to share positive observations while performing the task with the person in your care ('this is going well' or 'blood pressure is fine' or 'wound is nice and clean'). Experienced nurses have often become good at this but, while you are still learning, it helps to bookend your activities with personal communication and announce when your focus is going to be on the task at hand. The patient will understand you need to concentrate. By announcing that something might hurt a bit, you make sure that this does not come as a surprise. You also validate the pain as normal and not a personal oddity. Typically, patients respond more strongly to unexpected events. This is why you ask for permission and explain what you will do, what it is for, and how it will be experienced. This generates a degree of **cognitive control** for the person. As we've established, 'regaining control' is an important aspect of the response to injury or illness and facilitates healing or recovery. If you need to communicate with a colleague as part of the tasks you perform, involve the patient in the verbal interaction.

Activity 10.9 *Communication*

Clio (16) has self-harmed. There are deep cuts in her arms. They need to be examined, disinfected, stitched, and the bleeding needs to be stopped. List the order of activities and consider your communication with Clio. Make use of the four psychological approaches discussed here. Address the likely concerns Clio may have.

An outline answer is provided at the end of the chapter.

Medication distribution

Mary Poppins sang 'Just a spoonful of sugar makes the medicine go down', a catchy song that illustrates an important principle of administering medication. With children it is evident that masking the natural taste of a particular medicine with sugar turns the potentially aversive experience into a reinforcing one. This behavioural principle ensures that we are thus conditioned from childhood onwards.

Interestingly, adult oral medication hardly ever makes use of appealing flavours. The challenge for nurses is to find other incentives. Just about any positive experience associated with swallowing a series of pills can serve as reinforcement. Nonetheless, the reality is that adherence to medication is often compromised when left to the patients themselves (Haynes *et al.*, 2008). Self-management of medication tends to lead to forgetting or reducing the dose about half of the time (Nieuwlaat *et al.*, 2014). A systematic review of efforts to address this, including education, family support, reinforcement, motivational interviewing and CBT, did not show consistent improvements (Haynes *et al.*, 2008; Nieuwlaat *et al.*, 2014). In a hospital you can stay with the patient to ensure medication has been taken. The problem is that this does not promote **self-directed adherence** outside of the hospital. The above suggests that nurses should pay extra attention to medication adherence through reinforcement, conditioning, reminders and other behavioural techniques, but also ensure that patients become intrinsically motivated and are prepared to take responsibility.

Another important aspect of administering medication is rooted in cognitive and positive psychology. You all know what the **placebo effect** is. You give people a pill with no active ingredients but tell them that it will have a particular impact. It is likely that a number of the people who took the pills will report that it worked. This effect is based on the expectations of the person and those who administer medication (Ogden, 2012). The nurse is in a position to affect these expectations by the way in which medication is presented. Research on the placebo effect is patchy as a recent systematic review demonstrates (Hróbjartsson and Gøtzsche, 2010), but the impact on pain and/or reported pain – the difference is not always clear – tended to hold up in several studies. Most importantly, if the placebo effect takes place with inert substances, it can also enhance the impact of active agents. Thus it would make sense for nurses and physicians to accompany medication with information and attitudes that enhance the patient's expectation of a positive impact.

Activity 10.10 *Communication*

Create a short introduction to pain medication for: (a) a highly educated adult; (b) an adult with limited education. Aim to maximise its motivating impact.

An outline answer is provided at the end of the chapter.

Emergency response

Providing cardiopulmonary resuscitation (CPR) and other emergency interventions is a matter of life and death and therefore stressful. The problem with CPR is that many nurses don't encounter it often enough to become confident at it. So, even with repeat training at regular intervals, nurses may get overwhelmed by the occasion and may not be able to control their 'nerves'. Because being over-activated may lead to mistakes (Arent and Landers, 2003; Yerkes and Dodson, 1908), it is important that nurses can apply cognitive and behavioural control, such as through positive thinking and activation reduction or relaxation techniques (Davis *et al.*, 2008).

Furthermore, it is important for nurses to know that the success rate of CPR attempts may be lower than hoped for (30 per cent or less) (Esibov *et al.*, 2015). But, even while knowing this, a failed CPR is deeply affecting, especially for a novice nurse, and can conceivably lead to a post-traumatic stress reaction over time. Hospitals tend to have debriefing and peer-supports in place in which all three psychological perspectives are used to prevent post-traumatic stress. To what extent a traumatic reaction can be averted by such interventions is still a matter of debate (Devilly, *et al.*, 2006).

Activity 10.11 *Communication*

A nursing student has just been involved in a failed CPR attempt and is shaken and upset. Consider what you can do to help your fellow nurse. Make explicit what you can do from a humanistic perspective, a cognitive and a behavioural perspective while making use of positive psychology.

An outline answer is provided at the end of the chapter.

Other activities

Developing and updating patient care plans, handover and record keeping

Care plans and handover need to embrace a bio-psycho-social perspective. Unless you document it, holistic care will not happen. Of course, record keeping has become more comprehensive and complex in recent years and computer-based documentation has often transformed health-care communication (Lavin, *et al.*, 2015). There is some concern that record keeping has become so time-consuming that it interferes with patient contact (Hendrich, *et al.*, 2008). Moreover, it is not unthinkable that meticulous record keeping hidden away in an office can become an escape from the hardship of emotional labour.

Interactions with the multi-disciplinary team (MDT)

Working effectively and harmoniously within the hospital context requires developing and maintaining good contact and friendships with colleagues. As we've outlined in Chapter 7, there is a tendency to relate mostly within one's own professional group (Westbrook, *et al.*, 2011). While this is not surprising, it is evident that health-care facilities work best when individuals reach out and develop good personal contacts with other health-care professionals. Mutual respect is based on demonstrating competence (behavioural) and knowledge (cognitive). The humanistic perspective tends to come in when developing close relationships with co-workers. It is important because smooth working relations tend to reduce stress and enhance patient care. Multi-disciplinary team meetings (in which increasingly well-educated nurses have an important role) provide opportunities to develop those relationships. Please be aware that meetings that put too much emphasis on conformity within the team are at risk of developing 'group think' (Janis, 1982). This can lead to critical voices not being heard, which can be a source of mistakes.

Mentoring and being mentored

Being mentored is perhaps your main concern if you are studying for a degree. To make the most of your placements and internships it is essential that you develop a good relationship with a mentor or preceptor. Those relationships develop using humanistic, behavioural and cognitive principles. Most simply stated, the humanistic element is essential in developing a relationship through showing respect, interest and affection, while behavioural principles are at the basis of shaping nursing behaviours and skills (use of modelling, praise, encouragement, etc.). Cognitive principles form the essence of how you transmit knowledge, attitudes, values and understanding of nursing and health-care practice. Observe how good mentors operate; one day you will be called on to mentor student nurses yourself.

Interactions with family and other visitors

Because most nursing work in hospitals is with the patient and not the family, most of your contact with family and visitors is short and in passing. Sometimes family members are involved in information meetings and decision making. Those meetings tend to benefit from efforts by nurses to make sure that family members feel welcome during their visits. Greetings and friendly interactions may be very important to visitors, who often feel overwhelmed, concerned, and ill at ease. A humanistic perspective in contact with family and other visitors is likely to strengthen the impression that their loved one is in good hands. Also, don't forget that family members are an important source of support at all stages of the crisis of illness. It is essential that they are involved in all cognitive and behavioural aspects of care and rehabilitation. The nurse plays a pivotal role in reinforcing that message and recruiting family to be an active part of the care process. Family is also an important source of information. It is often through conversations with families that the full bio-psycho-social context of the person's illness can be understood.

Hygiene and safety activities, non-nursing tasks

Several hygiene and safety activities, including hand washing, are daily nursing tasks. Infection control is perhaps one of the most important safety measures in the hospital and adherence to hand-washing regulations is essential. Research shows that hand-washing standards are still not optimal in even the best hospitals (Allegranzi *et al.*, 2013). Continuous behavioural and cognitive efforts aimed at promoting and shaping hand washing are attempting to change this, but all of these efforts are futile if staff are not sufficiently motivated or aware. Forgetting to do it is a main concern. Moreover, if there is not enough time or the infrastructure is deficient (absent, inoperable or faulty taps, empty or absent alcohol rub stations), hand-washing practices can easily erode to unacceptably low levels. It is essential to maintain awareness of this and report it whenever there is a problem.

A wide variety of non-nursing tasks such as transporting patients or arranging transport, delivering food trays, housekeeping duties, ordering supplies, etc. are also part of most nurses' daily activities. While perhaps unavoidable, there is evidence that this may take away from the quality of care (Bekker, *et al.*, 2015). Research within the UK has demonstrated that when there is time pressure, it is the emotional support of patients, patient education and updating of patient care plans that are most likely to be left undone, not the non-nursing tasks (Ball, *et al.*, 2013).

Critical reflection

Each of the different nursing tasks poses a different challenge. Being aware and ambitious in your application of psychology will help you become really good at each of them. We would recommend that you reflect critically by asking yourself the following questions:

- **Humanistic perspective**: Do I show enough empathy? Am I listening well enough? Do I take what my patients say seriously and do I support how they make important decisions for themselves?
- **Cognitive perspective**: What is the patient thinking? If this leads to excessive anxiety or low mood, what can I do to change this? How can I promote effective thinking in my patients?
- **Behavioural perspective**: How do I plan my efforts to shape a patient's health behaviour or rehabilitation? Am I encouraging effectively? How can I be an effective model?
- **Positive psychology perspective**: Do I generate a positive mood, optimism and hope in the people in my care?

Critical reflection also means to critically evaluate whether your actual work is consistent with standards, regulations and values (such as the six Cs: Care, Compassion, Competence, Communication, Courage and Commitment – see Cummings and Bennett, 2012). Moreover, when it is not, you have to adapt and improve your efforts, rather than seek justifications in defence of why your work is not up to the expected level. This means allowing yourself to feel the discomfort of cognitive dissonance (Chapter 6) and choose a behavioural response rather than a cognitive defence. In your transition from student nurse to professional you will encounter pressure to become an efficient cog in the wheels of operation in the health-care organisation you work for. It is very important that you do not abandon what you have learned about evidence-based care and critical reflection (Dahl and Eriksen, 2016; Zerwekh and Garneau, 2014). There are useful guidelines to reflect in a structured way, specifically for nurses (Rolfe, *et al.*, 2010).

Without critical reflection and without continuous attempts to monitor and improve care levels, we are prone to mindlessly go through our daily routine. This may feel very comfortable. We tend to like automated activity and the reduced cognitive load that comes with it. The problem is that we are endangering the lives of our patients in this way. In light of this, it is important to be vigilant and to interrupt the flow of automated activity to check and double check. Critical reflection is difficult because it can be unpleasant, but it has the function of safety valves or circuit breakers and is therefore an important aspect of how we maintain safety (Reason, 1993; Reason, *et al.*, 2006). Without it we are more prone to make mistakes, fail to recognise important problems or fall victim to the gradual decline in care levels, which we call **care erosion** (de Vries and Timmins,

2016a; Timmins and de Vries, 2014). Please keep reminding yourself that 'unexamined care will become careless'. Psychology is at the heart of preventing this and therefore essential to all nurses.

Activity 10.12 — *Critical thinking*

Revisit Nurse A and Nurse B: **person-centred** versus **task-oriented** nursing (Chapter 1 p. 7).

- **Nurse A** listens, shows empathy, takes time with each patient and family, expresses an interest in both the patient and family, and involves them in all decisions.
- **Nurse B** works efficiently, has her work done on time, instructs and advises patients, and avoids invading the privacy between patient and family.

With what you know now, consider an average day in nursing care and analyse how both nurses would make use of the four psychological perspectives highlighted in this chapter.

An outline answer is provided at the end of the chapter.

Chapter summary

- Humanistic psychology informs compassionate care and targets patient feelings. Expressing empathy is at the core of this. While empathy needs to be felt to be genuine, it is important for nurses to learn to balance the intensity of care emotions to avoid care fatigue.
- Behavioural psychology informs rehabilitation, health promotion and other aspects of patient behaviour. The effective use of encouragement, scaffolding support and modelling healthy behaviour are key aspects of good nursing.
- Cognitive psychology informs nursing efforts to help patients think effectively about their condition and treatment. This is aimed at attitude change, strengthening motivation and reducing stress levels.
- Positive psychology emphasises the use of optimism and stimulation in care to enhance the overall impact of psychology on nursing quality.
- Critical reflection on daily care activities should include the application of psychological principles, consistency between care levels and values and standards, and efforts to examine automated and overly task-oriented interpretations of care.

Activities: brief outline answers

Activity 10.1: Humanistic care in practice (see page 166)

Some of the dehumanising aspects are subtle and can easily be compensated for, but don't underestimate their impact. It helps to consider what your own response would be if you were on the receiving end.

Activity 10.2: Behavioural care in practice (see page 168)

It is essential to ensure that the person tries out the desired activity, even if it is just a minute aspect of it. Modelling and encouragement can be used to make this happen. Support, instruction and reinforcement should then be used to further shape the behaviour.

Activity 10.3: Cognitive approach in care (see page 168)

This may require a lengthy conversation or a moment of inspiration in which you manage just the right thing that helps the person change perspective. It helps to point out the self-fulfilling prophecy of negative expectations.

Activity 10.4: Example of combined application in care (see page 169)

1) cognitive and positive psychology; 2) humanistic; 3) humanistic; 4) cognitive and humanistic; 5) cognitive and humanistic; 6) cognitive and positive psychology; 7) cognitive, behavioural, and positive psychology.

Activity 10.5: Communication (see page 174)

We tend to give instructions that make sense to us. This is not right. The most certain way to ensure that instructions work is to let patients actively structure them and represent them in a way that works for them. Following this, test them.

Activity 10.6: Critical thinking (see page 174)

A good reason to be selective is when information is overwhelming or increases a person's stress levels, with negative implications for the prognosis. If you offer to give further information when requested at a later time this addresses part of the ethical problem.

Activity 10.7: Decision making (see page 176)

To check the zone of development for the three challenges you need a hands-on investigation of how much help is needed to perform them. On the basis of this you can adjust the exercise sequence and design your scaffolding plan.

Activity 10.8: Persuasion (see page 177)

Persuading someone to get out of bed requires cognitive and behavioural efforts (see Activities 10.1 and 10.2), but also humanistic and positive psychology. The better your relationship, the more likely it is you will have an impact.

Activity 10.9: Communication (see page 177)

While you might feel compelled to lecture Clio (cognitive) and give discouraging signals (behavioural), you need to realise that self-harm represents Clio's unheard voice. This requires a humanistic perspective (listening, unconditional regard, empathy) before anything else.

Activity 10.10: Communication (see page 178)

For example: (a) This pain medication has an 80 per cent success rate in reducing the pain by half and has very limited side-effects. It has been used with soldiers with battle injuries who considered it more effective than other pain medication. (b) I've used this too; it is great.

Activity 10.11: Communication (see page 179)

The core question is: is it good to talk? Do not continue when you sense that your colleague only gets more upset when talking. You can provide other humanistic support. Cognitive efforts could include giving information on how common CPR failure is. Behavioural efforts could involve going for a walk and, if your colleague is ready, revisit the room in which the CPR effort took place. Be sensitive to the needs of your colleague.

Activity 10.12: Critical thinking final activity (see page 182)

Evidently Nurse A will make more use of psychology than Nurse B. In particular, humanistic person-centred principles are not included by Nurse B. Nurse B may attempt to compensate with the use of optimism and energy (positive psychology). Nurse B-type care is more common when there are staff shortages and nurses have less time for patients.

Further reading

Upton, D. and Thirlaway, K. (2010) *Promoting healthy behaviour: a practical guide for nursing and healthcare professionals.* Harlow, UK: Pearson Education Limited.

This text provides practical guidance for the promotion of eating well, being active and how to kick bad habits.

Walker, S. (Ed.) (2015) *Psychosocial interventions in mental health nursing.* London, UK: Sage.

While this text is written for mental health nurses it is highly relevant to all nurses.

Marsh, H. (2014) *Do no harm: stories of life, death and brain surgery.* London, UK: Weidenfeld and Nicholson.

This candid account of the highs and lows in the life and practice of a neurosurgeon is a highlight of critically reflective practice.

Zerwekh, J. and Garneau, A. Z. (2014) *Nursing today: transition and trends.* Philadelphia, PA: Elsevier Health Sciences.

This well laid out American text addresses the transition from student to professional nurse and may broaden your horizons.

Rolfe, G., Jasper, M. and Freshwater, D. (2010) *Critical reflection in practice: generating knowledge for care* (2nd Ed.). Hampshire, UK: Palgrave Macmillan.

This text on critical reflection relates well to the principles we've outlined for the use of psychology in critical reflection.

Useful websites

http://www.who.int/mental_health/en/

World Health Organisation (WHO) webpages on mental health represent a global perspective on the relationship between health and psychology.

http://www.apa.org/pi/about/publications/caregivers/

The Caregiver Briefcase offers a professional psychological perspective on caregiving in the community and in health-care centres.

https://www.psychologytoday.com/basics/caregiving

Psychology Today is a magazine that offers online access. This link takes you to a series of articles with valuable advice for caregivers. Search the magazine for other interesting material.

https://www.youtube.com/watch?v=fZffBAefwUM

Ellen Langer 'Counterclockwise: the power of possibility' at Happiness and Its Causes 2012. This is one of her talks on Mindfulness with many references to health. There are several other ones.

References

Adler, H. (2002) *Handbook of NLP: a manual for professional communicators.* Aldershot, UK: Gower Publishing Ltd.

Ainsworth, M., Blehar, M., Waters, E. and Wall, S. (1978) *Patterns of attachment: observations in the strange situation and at home.* Hillsdale, NJ: Lawrence Erlbaum Associates, Inc.

Ainsworth, S. (1999) The functions of multiple representations. *Computers and Education,* 33(2): 131-152.

Akkerman, R. and Knape, J. (2014) [Waking up during general anaesthesia]. *Nederlands Tijdschrift voor Geneeskunde* 159: A8705-A8705.

Allegranzi, B., Gayet-Ageron, A., Damani, N., Bengaly, L., McLaws, M.-L., Moro, M.L. ... Storr, J. (2013) Global implementation of WHO's multimodal strategy for improvement of hand hygiene: a quasi-experimental study. *The Lancet Infectious Diseases,* 13(10): 843–851.

Anderson, L., Oldridge, N., Thompson, D. R., Zwisler, A.-D., Rees, K., Martin, N. and Taylor, R. S. (2016) Exercise-based cardiac rehabilitation for coronary heart disease: Cochrane systematic review and meta-analysis. *Journal of the American College of Cardiology,* 67: 1–12.

Arent, S. M. and Landers, D. M. (2003) Arousal, anxiety, and performance: a re-examination of the inverted-U hypothesis. *Research Quarterly for Exercise and Sport,* 74(4): 436–444.

Aronson, E. (1969) The theory of cognitive dissonance: a current perspective. *Advances in Experimental Social Psychology,* 4: 1–34.

Aronson, E. (2004) *The social animal* (9th Ed.). New York, NY: Worth.

Aronson, E. and Bridgeman, D. (1992) 'Jigsaw groups and the desegregated classroom: in pursuit of common goals' in E. Aronson (Ed.) *Readings on the social animal.* New York, NY: W. H. Freeman, pp. 430–440.

Asch, S. E. (1946) Forming impressions of personality. *The Journal of Abnormal and Social Psychology,* 41: 258.

Asch, S. E. (1956) Studies of independence and conformity: a minority of one against a unanimous majority. *Psychological Monographs,* 70: 70.

Atchley, R. C. (1980) *The social forces in later life: an introduction to social gerontology.* Belmont, CA: Wadsworth Publishing Company.

Atkinson, R. C. and Shiffrin, R. M. (1968) 'Human memory: a proposed system and its control processes' in Spence, K. W. and Spence, J. T. (Eds.) *The Psychology of Learning and Motivation.* New York: Academic Press.

Backs, R. W. and Seljos, K. A. (1994) Metabolic and cardiorespiratory measures of mental effort: the effects of level of difficulty in a working memory task. *International Journal of Psychophysiology,* 16: 57–68.

Baddeley, A. (2000) The episodic buffer: a new component of working memory? *Trends in Cognitive Sciences,* 4: 417–423.

Baddeley, A. and Hitch, G. J. (1974) Working memory. *The Psychology of Learning and Motivation,* 8: 47–89.

Baker, R. R. and Bellis, M. A. (1995) *Human sperm competition: copulation, masturbation and infidelity.* London: Chapman & Hall.

Ball, J. E., Murrells, T., Rafferty, A. M., Morrow, E. and Griffiths, P. (2013) 'Care left undone' during nursing shifts: associations with workload and perceived quality of care. *BMJ Quality and Safety,* bmjqs-2012-001767.

Baltes, P. B. and Baltes, M. M. (1990) Psychological perspectives on successful aging: the model of selective optimization with compensation. *Successful Aging: Perspectives from the Behavioral Sciences,* 1: 1–34.

Baltes, M. M. and Skinner, E. A. (1983) Cognitive performance deficits and hospitalization: learned helplessness, instrumental passivity or what? Comment on Raps, Peterson, Jonas, and Seligman. *Journal of Personality and Social Psychology,* Vol 45(5): 1013–1016.

Bandman, E. L. and Bandman, B. (1988) *Critical thinking in nursing.* San Mateo, CA: McGraw-Hill/Appleton and Lange.

Bandura, A., Ross, D. and Ross, S. A. (1963) Imitation of film-mediated aggressive models. *The Journal of Abnormal and Social Psychology,* 66: 3.

Barnes, D. E. and Yaffe, K. (2011) The projected effect of risk factor reduction on Alzheimer's disease prevalence. *The Lancet Neurology,* 10: 819–828.

Bastian, B. and Haslam, N. (2010) Excluded from humanity: the dehumanizing effects of social ostracism. *Journal of Experimental Social Psychology,* 46(1): 107–113.

Baumrind, D. (1971) Current patterns of parental authority. *Developmental Psychology,* 4: 1.

Bedwell, W. L., Wildman, J. L., Diazgranados, D., Salazar, M., Kramer, W. S. and Salas, E. (2012) Collaboration at work: an integrative multilevel conceptualization. *Human Resource Management Review,* 22: 128–145.

Becker, G. and Newsom, E. (2005) Resilience in the face of serious illness among chronically ill African Americans in later life. *The Journals of Gerontology Series B: Psychological Sciences and Social Sciences,* 60: 214–223.

Bekker, M., Coetzee, S. K., Klopper, H. C. and Ellis, S. M. (2015) Non-nursing tasks, nursing tasks left undone and job satisfaction among professional nurses in South African hospitals. *Journal of Nursing Management,* 23(8): 1115–1125.

Belloc, N. B. (1973) Relationship of health practices and mortality. *Preventive Medicine,* 2: 67–81.

Belloc, N. B. and Breslow, L. (1972) Relationship of physical health status and health practices. *Preventive Medicine,* 1: 409–421.

Benjamin, A. S. (2010) Representational explanations of "process" dissociations in recognition: the DRYAD theory of aging and memory judgments. *Psychological Review,* 117: 1055.

Bergenthal, N., Will, A., Streckmann, F., Wolkewitz, K. D., Monsef, I., Engert, A., Elter, T. and Skoetz, N. (2014) Aerobic physical exercise for adult patients with haematological malignancies. *Cochrane Database of Systematic Reviews,* 11.

Bernhofer, E. I., Higgins, P. A., Daly, B. J., Burant, C. J. and Hornick, T. R. (2014) Hospital lighting and its association with sleep, mood and pain in medical inpatients. *Journal of Advanced Nursing*, 70: 1164–1173.

Bernstein, D. A., Clarke-Stewart, A., Penner, L. A. and Roy, E. J. (2012) *Psychology* (9th Ed., Int. version). Belmont, CA: Wadsworth (Cengage Learning).

Berscheid, E. and Walster, E. (1974) 'Physical attractiveness' in L. Berkowitz (Ed.) *Advances in Experimental Social Psychology*, Volume 7, pp. 157–215.

Bienvenu, O., Gellar, J., Althouse, B., Colantuoni, E., Sricharoenchai, T., Mendez-Tellez, P., Shanholtz, C., Dennison, C., Pronovost, P. and Needham, D. (2013) Post-traumatic stress disorder symptoms after acute lung injury: a 2-year prospective longitudinal study. *Psychological Medicine*, 43: 2657–2671.

Biller-Andorno, N. and Zeltner, T. (2015) Individual responsibility and community solidarity – the Swiss health care system. *New England Journal of Medicine*, 373, 2193–2197.

Bin, Y. S., Marshall, N. S. and Glozier, N. (2012) Secular trends in adult sleep duration: a systematic review. *Sleep Medicine Reviews*, 16: 223–230.

Bower, G. H. (1981) Mood and memory. *American Psychologist*, 36: 129.

Bower, G. H. (1991) 'Mood congruity of social judgments' in J. P. Forgas (Ed.) *Emotion and social judgments* (pp. 31–54). Oxford, UK: Pergamon.

Bowlby, J. (2005) *A secure base: clinical applications of attachment theory*. Abingdon, UK: Taylor & Francis.

BPS (2015) *Division of Clinical Psychology: Mission Statement* [Online]. British Psychological Society. Available at: http://www.bps.org.uk/networks-and-communities/member-microsite/division-clinical-psychology (accessed 26 June 2015).

Brehm, S. S. and Brehm, J. W. (2013) *Psychological reactance: a theory of freedom and control*. Cambridge, MA: Academic Press.

Bremmer, J. N. (1987) Romulus, Remus and the foundation of Rome. *Roman Myth and Mythography*, pp. 25–48.

Breslow, L. and Enstrom, J. E. (1980) Persistence of health habits and their relationship to mortality. *Preventive Medicine*, 9: 469–483.

Brown, D. (2015) Health promotion in multicultural populations: a handbook for practitioners and students. *Health Promotion Practice*, 16(5): 629–630.

Brown, R. A., Abrantes, A. M., Minami, H., Read, J. P., Marcus, B. H., Jakicic, J. M., Strong, D. R., Dubreuil, M. E., Gordon, A. A. and Ramsey, S. E. (2014) A preliminary, randomized trial of aerobic exercise for alcohol dependence. *Journal of Substance Abuse Treatment*, 47: 1–9.

Brownell, K. D. and Rodin, J. (1994) The dieting maelstrom: is it possible and advisable to lose weight? *American Psychologist*, 49: 781.

Burger, J. M. (2009) Replicating Milgram: would people still obey today? *American Psychologist*, 64: 1.

Burr, C. B. (1906) *A primer of psychology and mental disease: for use in training schools for attendants and nurses and in medical classes and as a ready reference for the practitioner* (3rd Ed.). Philadelphia, PA: F.A. Davis Co.

Buss, D. M. (1999) *Evolutionary psychology: the new science of the mind*. Boston, MA: Allyn & Bacon.

Buzan, Tony (2006) *Use your memory: understand your mind to improve your memory and mental power.* Harlow, UK: BBC Active, Pearson Education.

Cacioppo, J. T., Petty, R. E. and Losch, M. E. (1986) Attributions of responsibility for helping and doing harm: evidence for confusion of responsibility. *Journal of Personality and Social Psychology*, 50: 100–105.

Camacho, E. M., Verstappen, S. M., Chipping, J. and Symmons, D. P. (2013) Learned helplessness predicts functional disability, pain and fatigue in patients with recent-onset inflammatory polyarthritis. *Rheumatology*, 52: 1233–1238.

Cameron, L. D. and Leventhal, H. (2003) *The self-regulation of health and illness behaviour.* London, UK: Routledge (Taylor and Francis).

Cannon, W. B. (1935) Stresses and strains of homeostasis. *The American Journal of the Medical Sciences*, 189: 13–14.

Caplan, G. (1964) *Principles of preventive psychiatry.* New York, NY: Basic Books.

Care, T. (2012) *A national response to Winterbourne View Hospital.* Department of Health Review: Final Report.

Cartwright, R. D. (1974) Problem solving: waking and dreaming. *Journal of Abnormal Psychology*, 83: 451–455.

Carver, C. S., Scheier, M. F. and Segerstrom, S. C. (2010) Optimism. *Clinical Psychology Review*, 30: 879–889.

Castell, B. D., Kazantzis, N. and Moss-Morris, R. E. (2011) Cognitive behavioral therapy and graded exercise for chronic fatigue syndrome: a meta-analysis. *Clinical Psychology: Science and Practice*, 18: 311–324.

Cheng, C., Lau, H.-P. B. and Chan, M.-P. S. (2014) Coping flexibility and psychological adjustment to stressful life changes: a meta-analytic review. *Psychological Bulletin*, 140: 1582–1607.

Chou, T. L., Chang, L. I. and Chung, M. H. (2015) The mediating and moderating effects of sleep hygiene practice on anxiety and insomnia in hospital nurses. *International Journal of Nursing Practice*, 21: 9–18.

Chugani, H. T., Behen, M. E., Muzik, O., Juhász, C., Nagy, F. and Chugani, D. C. (2001) Local brain functional activity following early deprivation: a study of postinstitutionalized Romanian orphans. *Neuroimage*, 14: 1290–1301.

Cialdini, R. B., Vincent, J. E., Lewis, S. K., Catalan, J., Wheeler, D. and Darby, B. L. (1975) Reciprocal concessions procedure for inducing compliance: the door-in-the-face technique. *Journal of Personality and Social Psychology*, 31: 206–215.

Clancy, S. A., Schacter, D. L., McNally, R. J. and Pitman, R. K. (2000) False recognition in women reporting recovered memories of sexual abuse. *Psychological Science*, 11: 26–31.

Clark, D. (2002) Between hope and acceptance: the medicalisation of dying. *British Medical Journal*, 324: 905–907.

Cohen, M. A. and Dennett, D. C. (2011) Consciousness cannot be separated from function. *Trends in Cognitive Sciences*, 15: 358–364.

Commisso, M. and Finkelstein, L. (2012) Physical attractiveness bias in employee termination. *Journal of Applied Social Psychology*, 42: 2968–2987.

Compas, B. E., Jaser, S. S., Dunn, M. J. and Rodriguez, E. M. (2012) Coping with chronic illness in childhood and adolescence. *Annual Review of Clinical Psychology*, 8: 455–480.

Coon, D. (2004) Introduction to Psychology: Gateways to Mind and Behaviour (10th Ed.). Belmont, CA: Thomson-Wadsworth.

Coon, D. and Mitterer, J. (2012) *Introduction to psychology: gateways to mind and behavior with concept maps and reviews.* Andover, UK: Cengage Learning.

Cooper, J. (2007) *Cognitive dissonance: 50 years of a classic theory.* London, UK: Sage.

Cosmides, L. (1989) The logic of social exchange: has natural selection shaped how humans reason? Studies with the Wason selection task. *Cognition,* 31: 187–276.

Cosmides, L. and Tooby, J. (1992) 'Cognitive adaptations for social exchange' in J. H. Barkow, L. Cosmides and J. Tooby (Eds) *The adapted mind: evolutionary psychology and the generation of culture.* Oxford, UK: Oxford University Press.

Crawford, F. A., Mammon, J. W. and Shingleton, W. W. (1971) The stress ulcer syndrome: a clinical and pathologic review. *The American Journal of Surgery,* 121: 644–649.

Crum, A. J., Salovey, P. and Achor, S. (2013) Rethinking stress: the role of mindsets in determining the stress response. *Journal of Personality and Social Psychology,* 104: 716–733.

Cumming, E., Henry, W. E. and Damianopoulos, E. (1961) 'A formal statement of disengagement theory' in E. Cumming and W. E. Henry *Growing old: the process of disengagement.* New York, NY: Basic Books, pp. 210–218.

Cummings, J. and Bennett, V. (2012) *Compassion in practice: nursing, midwifery and care staff: our vision and strategy.* Online, last accessed on 23 July 2014. Available at: http://www. england. nhs. uk/wp-content/ uploads/2012/12/compassion-inpractice.pdf

Dahl, H. and Eriksen, K. Å. (2016) Students' and teachers' experiences of participating in the reflection process "THiNK". *Nurse Education Today,* 36: 401–406.

Damasio, A., Meyer, K., Laureys, S. and Tononi, G. (2009) 'Consciousness: an overview of the phenomenon and of its possible neural basis' in S. Laureys and G. Tononi (Eds) *The Neurology of Consciousness: Cognitive Neuroscience and Neuropathology,* pp. 3–14.

Darbyshire, P. (2014) Character assassination? Response to John Paley "social psychology and the compassion deficit". *Nurse Education Today,* 34: 887–889.

Darley, J. M. and Latané, B. (1968) Bystander intervention in emergencies: diffusion of responsibility. *Journal of Personality and Social Psychology,* 8: 377–381.

Darwin, C. (1859) *On the origin of species by means of natural selection.* London, UK: Murray.

Davies, P. G., Spencer, S. J. and Steele, C. M. (2005) Clearing the air: identity safety moderates the effects of stereotype threat on women's leadership aspirations. *Journal of Personality and Social Psychology,* 88: 276–287.

Davis, M., Eshelman, E. R. and McKay, M. (2008) *The relaxation and stress reduction workbook.* Oakland, CA: New Harbinger Publications.

Davis, S. W., Dennis, N. A., Daselaar, S. M., Fleck, M. S. and Cabeza, R. (2008) Que PASA? The posterior–anterior shift in aging. *Cerebral cortex,* 18: 1201–1209.

Davydow, D. S., Zatzick, D., Hough, C. L. and Katon, W. J. (2013) A longitudinal investigation of posttraumatic stress and depressive symptoms over the course of the year following medical–surgical intensive care unit admission. *General Hospital Psychiatry*, 35: 226–232.

Dawkins, R. (2006) *The selfish gene.* Oxford, UK: Oxford University Press.

Dennett, D. C. (1993) *Consciousness explained.* London, Penguin.

Denzin, N. K. and Lincoln, Y. S. (2011) *The Sage handbook of qualitative research* (4th Ed.). London: Sage.

De Ridder, D., Geenen, R., Kuijer, R. and Van Middendorp, H. (2008) Psychological adjustment to chronic disease. *The Lancet*, 372: 246–255.

Devilly, G. J., Gist, R. and Cotton, P. (2006) Ready! Fire! Aim! The status of psychological debriefing and therapeutic interventions: in the work place and after disasters. *Review of General Psychology*, 10(4): 318–345.

De Vries, J. M. and Timmins, F. (2012) Psychology teaching in nursing education: a review of and reflection on approaches, issues, and contemporary practice. *Nurse Education in Practice* 12: 316–21.

De Vries, J. and Timmins, F. (2016a) Care erosion in hospitals: Problems in reflective nursing practice and the role of cognitive dissonance. *Nurse Education Today*, 38: 5–8.

De Vries, J. and Timmins, F. (2016b) Deception and self-deception in health care. *Nursing Philosophy*, 17: 163–172.

DiCenso, A., Bourgeault, I., Abelson, J., Martin-Misener, R., Kaasalainen, S., Carter, N., Harbman, P., Donald, F., Bryant-Lukosius, D. and Kilpatrick, K. (2010) Utilization of nurse practitioners to increase patient access to primary healthcare in Canada – thinking outside the box. *Nursing Leadership* (Toronto, Ont.), 23: 239–259.

Diehl, D. J. and Gershon, S. (1992) The role of dopamine in mood disorders. *Comprehensive Psychiatry*, 33: 115–120.

Dinsmore, D. L. and Alexander, P. A. (2012) A critical discussion of deep and surface processing: what it means, how it is measured, the role of context, and model specification. *Educational Psychology Review*, 24: 499–567.

Dion, K., Berscheid, E. and Walster, E. (1972) What is beautiful is good. *Journal of Personality and Social Psychology*, 24: 285–290.

Dittman, M. (2002) Study ranks the top 20th century psychologists. *Monitor on Psychology*, 33: 28–29.

Donovan, K. A., McGinty, H. L. and Jacobsen, P. B. (2013) A systematic review of research using the diagnostic criteria for cancer-related fatigue. *Psycho-Oncology*, 22: 737–744.

Dror, O. E. (2014) The Cannon–Bard thalamic theory of emotions: a brief genealogy and reappraisal. *Emotion Review*, 6: 13–20.

Dungan, J., Waytz, A. and Young, L. (2015) The psychology of whistleblowing. *Current Opinion in Psychology*, 6: 129–133.

Eccleston, C., Hearn, L. and Williams, A. (2015) Psychological therapies for the management of chronic neuropathic pain in adults. *Cochrane Database of Systematic Reviews* Oct 29;(10): CD011259. doi: 10.1002/14651858.CD011259.pub2.

Edinger, J. D., Bonnet, M. H., Bootzin, R. R., Doghramji, K., Dorsey, C. M., Espie, C. A., Jamieson, A. O., McCall, W. V., Morin, C. M. and Stepanski, E. J. (2004) Derivation of research diagnostic criteria for insomnia: report of an American Academy of Sleep Medicine Work Group. *Sleep*, 27: 1567–1596.

Eisenberger, N. I. and Lieberman, M. D. (2004) Why rejection hurts: a common neural alarm system for physical and social pain. *Trends in Cognitive Sciences*, 8: 294–300.

Ekman, P. (1992) An argument for basic emotions. *Cognition and Emotion*, 6: 169–200.

Ekman, P. and Friesen, W. V. (1971) Constants across cultures in the face and emotion. *Journal of Personality and Social Psychology*, 17: 124–129.

Ekman, P., Friesen, W. V., O'Sullivan, M., Chan, A., Diacoyanni-Tarlatzis, I., Heider, K., Krause, R., Lecompte, W. A., Pitcairn, T. and Ricci-Bitti, P. E. (1987) Universals and cultural differences in the judgments of facial expressions of emotion. *Journal of Personality and Social Psychology*, 53: 712–717.

Eliason, M. J. (1993) AIDS-related stigma and homophobia: implications for nursing education. *Nurse Educator*, 18: 27–30.

Eling, P., Aleman, A. and Krabbendam, L. (Eds.) (2013) *Cognitieve Neuropsychiatrie: een processbenadering van symptomen.* Amsterdam, NL: Boom.

Erickson, K. I., Weinstein, A. M. and Lopez, O. L. (2012) Physical activity, brain plasticity, and Alzheimer's disease. *Archives of Medical Research*, 43: 615–621.

Erikson, E. H. (1959) *Identity and the life cycle: selected papers: Psychological Issues, Vol. 1, No. 1.* New York, NY: International Universities Press, Inc.

Esibov, A., Banville, I., Chapman, F. W., Boomars, R., Box, M. and Rubertsson, S. (2015) Mechanical chest compressions improved aspects of CPR in the LINC trial. *Resuscitation*, 91: 116–121.

Ezzati, M. and Riboli, E. (2013) Behavioral and dietary risk factors for noncommunicable diseases. *New England Journal of Medicine*, 369: 954–964.

Federenko, I. S. and Wadhwa, P. D. (2004) Women's mental health during pregnancy influences fetal and infant developmental and health outcomes. *CNS Spectrums*, 9: 198–206.

Fenton, L. (2004) Preventing HIV/AIDS through poverty reduction: the only sustainable solution? *The Lancet*, 364: 1186–1187.

Festinger, L. (1957) *A theory of cognitive dissonance.* Stanford, CA: Stanford University Press.

Fiedler, K., Nickel, S., Muehlfriedel, T. and Unkelbach, C. (2001) Is mood congruency an effect of genuine memory or response bias? *Journal of Experimental Social Psychology*, 37: 201–214.

Firth-Cozens, J. and Greenhalgh, J. (1997) Doctors' perceptions of the links between stress and lowered clinical care. *Social Science and Medicine*, 44: 1017–1022.

Fiske, S. T. and Taylor, S. E. (1991) *Social cognition* (2nd Ed.). New York, NY: McGraw-Hill.

Fiske, S. T. (2000) Stereotyping, prejudice, and discrimination at the seam between the centuries: evolution, culture, mind, and brain. *European Journal of Social Psychology*, 30: 299–322.

Fiske, S. T. (2004) Intent and ordinary bias: Unintended thought and social motivation create casual prejudice. *Social Justice Research*, 17: 117–127.

Fletcher, G. F., Balady, G., Blair, S. N., Blumenthal, J., Caspersen, C., Chaitman, B., Epstein, S., Froelicher, E. S. S., Froelicher, V. F. and Pina, I. L. (1996) Statement on exercise: benefits and recommendations for physical activity programs for all Americans. A statement for health professionals by the committee on exercise and cardiac rehabilitation of the council on clinical cardiology (American Heart Association). *Circulation*, 94: 857–862.

Flinn, M. V., Geary, D. C. and Ward, C. V. (2005) Ecological dominance, social competition, and coalitionary arms races: why humans evolved extraordinary intelligence. *Evolution and Human Behavior*, 26: 10–46.

Forbes, J. E. (1919) Psychology for nurses. *The American Journal of Nursing*, 19: 6.

Fraga, A. (2015) Pretty probationers: the relationship between physical attractiveness and sentencing outcomes. The Ohio State University (electronic thesis or dissertation). Retrieved from https://etd.ohiolink.edu/

Frank, A. W. (2013) *The wounded storyteller: Body, illness, and ethics.* Chicago, IL: University of Chicago Press.

Freud, S. and Brill, A. A. (1916) *Wit and its relation to the unconscious.* Courier Corporation.

Freud, S. (1922) The unconscious. *The Journal of Nervous and Mental Disease*, 56: 291–294.

Freud, S. (1940) *Moses and Monotheism, an outline of psycho-analysis and other works (1937–1939): the development of the sexual function*, Standard Ed., Vol 23. London, UK: Hogarth Press and the Institute of Psychoanalysis(pp. 52–156).

Freud, S. (2010) *The interpretation of dreams.* New York, NY: Basic Books.

Friedman, M. and Rosenman, R. H. (1959) Association of specific overt behavior pattern with blood and cardiovascular findings: blood cholesterol level, blood clotting time, incidence of arcus senilis, and clinical coronary artery disease. *Journal of the American Medical Association*, 169: 1286–1296.

Frijda, N. (1986) *The emotions.* Cambridge, UK: Cambridge University Press.

Frodl, T. and O'Keane, V. (2013) How does the brain deal with cumulative stress? A review with focus on developmental stress, HPA axis function and hippocampal structure in humans. *Neurobiology of Disease*, 52: 24–37.

Garcia, A. W. and King, A. C. (1991) Predicting long-term adherence to aerobic exercise: a comparison of two models. *Journal of Sport and Exercise Psychology*, 13: 394–410.

Gardner, H. (2008) *The mind's new science: a history of the cognitive revolution.* New York, NY: Basic Books.

Gaulin, S. J. and McBurney, D. H. (2001) *Psychology: an evolutionary approach.* Upper Saddle River, NJ: Prentice Hall.

Gergen, K. J. and Gergen, M. (2010) 'Positive aging: resilience and reconstruction' in P. S. Fry and C. L. M. Keyes *New frontiers in resilient aging: life-strengths and well-being in late life.* Cambridge, UK: Cambridge University Press.

Gibson, E. J. and Walk, R. D. (1960) The "visual cliff". *Scientific American*, 202: 67–71.

Goffman, E. (1963) *Stigma: notes on the management of spoiled identity.* Englewood Cliffs, NJ: Prentice Hall Inc.

Goldenthal, P. (2000) Beyond sibling rivalry: how to help your children become cooperative, caring and compassionate. New York, NY: Henry Holt and Co.

Goleman, D. (1995) *Emotional intelligence.* New York, NY: Bantam Books.

Gonzalez-Liencres, C., Shamay-Tsoory, S. G. and Brüne, M. (2013) Towards a neuroscience of empathy: ontogeny, phylogeny, brain mechanisms, context and psychopathology. *Neuroscience and Biobehavioral Reviews,* 37(8): 1537–1548.

Grammer, K., Renninger, L. and Fischer, B. (2004) Disco clothing, female sexual motivation, and relationship status: is she dressed to impress? *Journal of Sex Research,* 41: 66–74.

Gray, B. (2012) *Face to face with emotions in health and social care.* New York, NY: Springer-Verlag.

Greenberg, D. J., Hillman, D. and Grice, D. (1973) Infant and stranger variables related to stranger anxiety in the first year of life. *Developmental Psychology,* 9: 207–212.

Gross, A. E. and Latané, J. G. (1974) Receiving help, reciprocation, and interpersonal attraction. *Journal of Applied Social Psychology,* 4: 210–223.

Gross, R. and Kinnison, N. (2014) *Psychology for Nurses and Allied Health Professionals: Applying Theory to Practice.* London: Routledge.

Guéguen, N. (2009) Menstrual cycle phases and female receptivity to a courtship solicitation: an evaluation in a nightclub. *Evolution and Human Behavior,* 30: 351–355.

Gupta, S. and Mittal, S. (2015) Runner's high: a review of the plausible mechanisms underlying exercise-induced ecstasy. *Saudi Journal of Sports Medicine,* 15: 207–209.

Hackett, M. L., Yapa, C., Parag, V. and Anderson, C. S. (2005) Frequency of depression after stroke: a systematic review of observational studies. *Stroke,* 36: 1330–1340.

Hagger, M. S. and Orbell, S. (2003) A meta-analytic review of the common-sense model of illness representations. *Psychology and Health,* 18: 141–184.

Hall, J. M., Podawiltz, A., Mummert, D. I., Jones, H. and Mummert, M. E. (2012) Psychological stress and the cutaneous immune response: roles of the HPA axis and the sympathetic nervous system in atopic dermatitis and psoriasis. *Dermatology Research and Practice* http://dx.doi.org/10.1371/journal.pone.0098283

Han, B. and Haley, W. E. (1999) Family caregiving for patients with stroke review and analysis. *Stroke,* 30: 1478–1485.

Hannigan, C., Coen, R. F., Lawlor, B. A., Robertson, I. H. and Brennan, S. (2015) The NEIL Memory Research Unit: psychosocial, biological, physiological and lifestyle factors associated with healthy ageing: study protocol. *BMC Psychology,* 20: 1–14.

Harris, R., Sims, S., Parr, J. and Davies, N. (2015) Impact of 12h shift patterns in nursing: a scoping review. *International Journal of Nursing Studies,* 52: 605–634.

Hasegawa, T. and Karandagoda, W. (2011) *Change management for hospitals. Through stepwise approach.* 5S-KAIZEN-TQM. Tokyo: JICA.

Haslam, S. A. and Reicher, S. D. (2012) Contesting the "nature" of conformity: what Milgram and Zimbardo's studies really show. *PLoS Biol* 10(11): e1001426.

Haynes, R. B., Ackloo, E., Sahota, N., McDonald, H. P. and Yao, X. (2008) Interventions for enhancing medication adherence. *Cochrane Database Syst Rev,* 2(2).

Heider, F. (1944) Social perception and phenomenal causality. *Psychological Review*, 51: 358–374.

Hendrich, A., Chow, M., Skierczynski, B. A. and Lu, Z. (2008) A 36-hospital time and motion study: how do medical-surgical nurses spend their time? *RCHE Publications*, 50: 25–34.

Heran, B. S., Chen, J., Ebrahim, S., Moxham, T., Oldridge, N., Rees, K., Thompson, D. R. and Taylor, R. S. (2011) Exercise-based cardiac rehabilitation for coronary heart disease. *Cochrane Database Syst Rev.*, 7.

Herring, M. P., Puetz, T. W., O'Connor, P. J. and Dishman, R. K. (2012) Effect of exercise training on depressive symptoms among patients with a chronic illness: a systematic review and meta-analysis of randomized controlled trials. *Archives of Internal Medicine*, 172: 101–111.

Heyes, A. (2005) The economics of vocation or 'why is a badly paid nurse a good nurse'? *Journal of Health Economics*, 24: 561–569.

Higgins, A. C. (1921) *The Psychology of Nursing*. New York and London: G.P. Putnam and Sons.

Hillman, C. H., Erickson, K. I. and Kramer, A. F. (2008) Be smart, exercise your heart: exercise effects on brain and cognition. *Nature Reviews Neuroscience*, 9: 58–65.

Hobfoll, S. E. and Freedy, J. (1993) *Conservation of resources: a general stress theory applied to burnout*. Abingdon, UK: Taylor & Francis.

Hodges, B. H. and Geyer, A. L. (2006) A nonconformist account of the Asch experiments: values, pragmatics, and moral dilemmas. *Personality and Social Psychology Review*, 10: 2–19.

Holmes, T. H. and Rahe, R. H. (1967) The social readjustment rating scale. *Journal of Psychosomatic Research*, 11: 213–218.

Hopkins, C. and MacKenzie, J. (2008) 'Crisis assessment and resolution' in: P. Barker (Ed.) *Psychiatric and mental health nursing: the craft of caring*. London, UK: Hodder Arnold, p. 426.

Horsley, J. A., Absalom, K. A., Akiens, E. M., Dunk, R. J. and Ferguson, A. M. (2014) The proportion of unhealthy foodstuffs children are exposed to at the checkout of convenience supermarkets. *Public Health Nutrition*, 17: 2453–2458.

Hosoda, M., Stone-Romero, E. F. and Coats, G. (2003) The effects of physical attractiveness on job-related outcomes: a meta-analysis of experimental studies. *Personnel Psychology*, 56: 431–462.

House, J. S. (1974) Occupational stress and coronary heart disease: a review and theoretical integration. *Journal of Health and Social Behavior*, 12–27.

Hróbjartsson, A. and Gøtzsche, P. C. (2010) Placebo interventions for all clinical conditions. *Cochrane Database Syst Rev*, 1(1).

Hsu, M.-Y. (2015) A Quality of Working Life Survey Instrument for hospital nurses. *The Journal of Nursing Research* (*JNR*), Mar; 24(1): 87–99.

Hudson, R. and Trillmich, F. (2008) Sibling competition and cooperation in mammals: challenges, developments and prospects. *Behavioral Ecology and Sociobiology*, 62: 299–307.

Huguet, A., McGrath, P. J., Stinson, J., Tougas, M. E. and Doucette, S. (2014) Efficacy of psychological treatment for headaches: an overview of systematic reviews and analysis of potential modifiers of treatment efficacy. *The Clinical Journal of Pain*, 30: 353–369.

Hull, C. L. (1943) *Principles of behaviour.* New York, NY: Appleton–Century-Crofts.

Hultsch, D. F., Hertzog, C., Small, B. J. and Dixon, R. A. (1999) Use it or lose it: engaged lifestyle as a buffer of cognitive decline in aging? *Psychology and Aging,* 14: 245–263.

Ikoma, A., Steinhoff, M., Ständer, S., Yosipovitch, G. and Schmelz, M. (2006) The neurobiology of itch. *Nature Reviews Neuroscience,* 7: 535–547.

Irwin, B. C., Scorniaenchi, J., Kerr, N. L., Eisenmann, J. C. and Feltz, D. L. (2012) Aerobic exercise is promoted when individual performance affects the group: a test of the Kohler motivation gain effect. *Annals of Behavioral Medicine,* 44: 151–159.

Izard, C. E. (1992) Basic emotions, relations among emotions, and emotion-cognition relations. *Psychological Review,* Jul; 99(3): 561–566.

Jackson, M., Harrison, P., Swinburn, B. and Lawrence, M. (2015) 'Marketing ethics in context: the promotion of unhealthy foods and beverages to children', Chapter 17 in A. Nill (Ed.) *Handbook on Ethics and Marketing.* Cheltenham, UK: Edward Elgar Publishing, p. 354.

James, N. (1989) Emotional labour: skill and work in the social regulation of feelings. *The Sociological Review,* 37(1): 15–42.

James, W. (1890) *The principles of psychology.* New York, NY: H. Holt and Company.

James, W. (1884) II.—What is an emotion? *Mind,* 188–205.

Janis, I. L. (1958) Psychological stress: psychoanalytic and behavioral studies of surgical patients. New York, NY: John Wiley and Sons.

Janis, I. L. (1982) *Groupthink: psychological studies of policy decisions and fiascos.* Boston, MA: Houghton Mifflin.

Janssen, P. P., De Jonge, J. and Bakker, A. B. (1999) Specific determinants of intrinsic work motivation, burnout and turnover intentions: a study among nurses. *Journal of Advanced Nursing,* 29: 1360–1369.

Jasper, M. (2013) *Beginning reflective practice* (2nd Ed.). Andover, UK: Cengage Learning.

Jaynes, J. (2000) *The origin of consciousness in the breakdown of the bicameral mind.* Boston, MA: Houghton Mifflin Harcourt.

Jobin, J., Wrosch, C. and Scheier, M. F. (2014) Associations between dispositional optimism and diurnal cortisol in a community sample: when stress is perceived as higher than normal. *Health Psychology,* 33(4): 382–391.

Joinson, C. (1992) Coping with compassion fatigue. *Nursing,* 22(4): 116–118.

Jones, E. E. and Nisbett, R. E. (1971) 'The actor and the observer: divergent perceptions of the causes of behavior' in E. E. Jones, D. E. Kanouse, H. H. Kelly, R.E. Nisbett, S. Valins and B. Weiner, (Eds) *Attribution: perceiving the causes of behaviour.* Morristown, NJ: General Learning Press.

Jones, F. and Riazi, A. (2011) Self-efficacy and self-management after stroke: a systematic review. *Disability and rehabilitation,* 33: 797–810.

Josephson, B. R. (1996) Mood regulation and memory: repairing sad moods with happy memories. *Cognition and Emotion,* 10: 437–444.

Kagan, J., Reznick, J. S. and Snidman, N. (1988) Biological bases of childhood shyness. *Science,* 240: 167–171.

Kahneman, D. (2011) *Thinking, fast and slow.* London, UK: Penguin.

Kaiser, L. and Allen, L. H. (2008) Position of the American Dietetic Association: nutrition and lifestyle for a healthy pregnancy outcome. *J. Am Diet Assoc,* 108: 553–561.

Kanter, P. F., Medrano, L. and Conn, H. (2015) Does mood affect self-concept? Analysis through a natural semantic networks based approach. *International Journal of Behavioral Research and Psychology,* 3: 114–120.

Katz, J. and Rosenbloom, B. (2015) The Golden Anniversary of Melzack and Wall's gate control theory of pain: celebrating fifty years of pain research and management. *Pain Research and Management* Nov-Dec; 20(6): 285–291.

Kehyayan, V., Hirdes, J. P., Tyas, S. L. and Stolee, P. (2015) Residents' self-reported quality of life in long-term care facilities in Canada. *Canadian Journal on Aging/La Revue canadienne du vieillissement,* 34: 149–164.

Kelly, D. and Smith, P. (2016) 'Caring, face-work and nursing' (Ch 5) in H. Allan, M. Traynor, D. Kelly and P. Smith (Eds) *Understanding Sociology in Nursing.* London, UK: Sage.

Kennedy, P., Lude, P., Elfström, M. and Smithson, E. (2010) Cognitive appraisals, coping and quality of life outcomes: a multi-centre study of spinal cord injury rehabilitation. *Spinal Cord,* 48: 762–769.

Kitzinger, S. (2006) *Birth crisis.* London and New York: Routledge.

Kobasa, S. C. (1982) Commitment and coping in stress resistance among lawyers. *Journal of Personality and Social Psychology,* 42(4): 707–717.

Kobasa, S. C., Maddi, S. R. and Puccetti, M. C. (1982) Personality and exercise as buffers in the stress-illness relationship. *Journal of Behavioral Medicine,* 5: 391–404.

Koffka, K. (1921) *Die grundlagen der psychischen entwicklung.* Osterwieck AM Harz: Verlag Von A. W. Zickfeldt.

Kohlberg, L. (1984) *The psychology of moral development: the nature and validity of moral stages.* New York, NY: Harper Collins College Division.

Kok, L., Hillegers, M. H., Veldhuijzen, D. S., Cornelisse, S., Nierich, A. P., Van Der Maaten, J. M., Rosseel, P. M., Hofland, J., Sep, M. S. and Dieleman, J. M. (2015) The effect of Dexamethasone on symptoms of posttraumatic stress disorder and depression after cardiac surgery and intensive care admission: longitudinal follow-up of a randomized controlled trial. *Critical Care Medicine,* Mar; 44(3): 512–520.

Konok, V., Nagy, K. and Miklósi, Á. (2015) How do humans represent the emotions of dogs? The resemblance between the human representation of the canine and the human affective space. *Applied Animal Behaviour Science,* 162: 37–46.

Kosco, M. and Warren, N. A. (2000) Critical care nurses' perceptions of family needs as met. *Critical Care Nursing Quarterly,* 23: 60–72.

Kosfeld, M. (2007) *Trust in the brain.* EMBO Reports, 8: 44–47.

Kübler-Ross, E. (1969) *On death and dying.* New York, NY: Macmillan, pp. 45–9.

Kundera, M. (1996) *Laughable loves.* London, UK: Faber and Faber.

Kwakkel, G., Van Peppen, R., Wagenaar, R. C., Dauphinee, S. W., Richards, C., Ashburn, A., Miller, K., Lincoln, N., Partridge, C. and Wellwood, I. (2004) Effects of augmented exercise therapy time after stroke: a meta-analysis. *Stroke,* 35: 2529–2539.

Lachman, V. D. (2001) Professional presence: how do you get it? *Nursing Management*, 32(10): 41.

Lancaster, G. I. and Febbraio, M. A. (2015) Exercise and the immune system: implications for elite athletes and the general population. *Immunology and Cell Biology*, 94: 115–116.

Langer, E., Djikic, M., Pirson, M., Madenci, A. and Donohue, R. (2010) Believing is seeing using mindlessness (mindfully) to improve visual acuity. *Psychological Science*, May; 21(5): 661–667.

Langer, E. J., Janis, I. L. and Wolfer, J. A. (1975) Reduction of psychological stress in surgical patients. *Journal of Experimental Social Psychology*, 11(2): 155–165.

Langer, E. J. and Moldoveanu, M. (2000) The construct of mindfulness. *Journal of Social Issues*. 56: 1–9.

Latané, B. and Darley, J. M. (1969) Bystander "Apathy". *American Scientist*, 57(2): 244–268.

Latané, B. and Nida, S. (1981) Ten years of research on group size and helping. *Psychological Bulletin*, 89(2): 308–324.

Launiala, A. and Honkasalo, M. L. (2010) Malaria, danger, and risk perceptions among the Yao in rural Malawi. *Medical Anthropology Quarterly*, 24: 399–420.

Laureys, S. and Tononi, G. (2011) *The neurology of consciousness: cognitive neuroscience and neuropathology*. Cambridge, MA: Academic Press.

Lavin, M., Harper, E. and Barr, N. (2015) Health information technology, patient safety, and professional nursing care documentation in acute care settings. *OJIN: The Online Journal of Issues in Nursing*, 20(2).

Lazarus, R. S. and Folkman, S. (1984) *Stress, appraisal, and coping*. New York, NY: Springer.

Leiter, M. P. and Maslach, C. (2009) Nurse turnover: the mediating role of burnout. *Journal of Nursing Management*, 17: 331–339.

Leknes, S. and Tracey, I. (2008) A common neurobiology for pain and pleasure. *Nature Reviews Neuroscience*, 9: 314–320.

Leventhal, H., Brissette, I. and Leventhal, E. A. (2003) 'The common-sense model of self-regulation of health and illness' in L. D. Cameron and H. Leventhal (Eds) *The Self-Regulation of Health and Illness Behaviour*. London, UK: Routledge, p. 42–65.

Leventhal, H., Meyer, D. and Nerenz, D. (1980) The common sense representation of illness danger' in S. Rachman (Ed.) *Contributions to Medical Psychology*, Vol. 2. New York, NY: Pergamon Press, pp. 7–30.

Lewin, K. (1935) *A dynamic theory of personality*. New York, NY: McGraw-Hill.

Lewis, M. D. (2002) 'Interacting time scales in personality (and cognitive) development: Intentions, emotions, and emergent forms' in N. Granott and J. Parziale (Eds.) *Microdevelopment: transition processes in development and learning*. pp. 183–212. Cambridge Studies in Cognitive and Perceptual Development. (No. 7). Cambridge, UK: Cambridge University Press.

Leyendecker, B., Lamb, M. E., Fracasso, M. P., Schölmerich, A. and Larson, C. (1997) Playful interaction and the antecedents of attachment: a longitudinal study of Central American and Euro-American mothers and infants. *Merrill-Palmer Quarterly (1982-)*, 24–47.

Lin, F. R., Metter, E. J., O'Brien, R. J., Resnick, S. M., Zonderman, A. B. and Ferrucci, L. (2011) Hearing loss and incident dementia. *Archives of Neurology*, 68: 214–220.

Littlewood, D. L., Gooding, P. A., Panagioti, M. and Kyle, S. D. (2015) Nightmares and suicide in post-traumatic stress disorder: the mediating role of defeat, entrapment, and hopelessness. *Journal of Clinical Sleep Medicine*, March;12(3): 393–9 *JCSM [Official Publication of the American Academy of Sleep Medicine]*.

Loftus, E. and Ketcham, K. (1996) *The myth of repressed memory: false memories and allegations of sexual abuse.* London, UK: Macmillan Publishers.

Loftus, E. F. (1996) *Eyewitness testimony.* Cambridge, MA: Harvard University Press.

Loftus, E. F. (2005) Planting misinformation in the human mind: a 30-year investigation of the malleability of memory. *Learning & Memory*, 12: 361–366.

London, K., Bruck, M., Ceci, S. J. and Shuman, D. W. (2005) Disclosure of child sexual abuse: what does the research tell us about the ways that children tell? *Psychology, Public Policy, and Law*, 11(1): 194–226.

Lorber, J. (1975) Good patients and problem patients: conformity and deviance in a general hospital. *Journal of Health and Social Behavior*, 213–225.

Lorenz, K. (1937) (on imprinting) The companion in the bird's world. *Auk*, 54: 245–73.

Lowry, R. (1971) *The evolution of psychological theory: 1650 to present.* Chicago, IL: Aldine.

Maccoby, E. E. (1992) The role of parents in the socialization of children: an historical overview. *Developmental Psychology*, 28(6): 1006–1017.

MacLennan, B. (1996) The elements of consciousness and their neurodynamical correlates. *Journal of Consciousness Studies*, 3: 409–424.

MacLean, P. D. and Kral, V. A. (1973) *A triune concept of the brain and behaviour.* Published for the Ontario Mental Health Foundation by University of Toronto Press.

Manabe, K., Matsui, T., Yamaya, M., Sato-Nakagawa, T., Okamura, N., Arai, H. and Sasaki, H. (2000) Sleep patterns and mortality among elderly patients in a geriatric hospital. *Gerontology*, 46: 318–322.

Mannion, R. and Davies, H. T. (2015) Cultures of silence and cultures of voice: the role of whistleblowing in healthcare organisations. *International Journal of Health Policy and Management*, 4(8): 503–505.

Marcia, J. E. (1980) 'Identity in adolescence', Chapter 5 in J. Adelson (Ed.) *Handbook of Adolescent Psychology*, New York, NY: John Wiley, pp. 159–187.

Marks, D. F., Murray, M., Evans, B. and Estacio, E. V. (2011) *Health psychology: theory, research and practice* (3rd Ed.). London, UK: Sage.

Martin, P., Da Rosa, G., Siegler, I. C., Davey, A., MacDonald, M., Poon, L. W. and Study, G. C. (2006) Personality and longevity: findings from the Georgia Centenarian Study. *Age*, 28: 343–352.

Maslach, C. (2003) *Burnout: the cost of caring.* Cambridge, MA: Malor Books.

Maslach, C., Schaufeli, W. B. and Leiter, M. P. (2001) Job burnout. *Annual Review of Psychology*, 52: 397–422.

Maslow, A. H. (1943) A theory of human motivation. *Psychological Review*, 50(4): 370–396.

Maslow, A. H., Frager, R., Fadiman, J., McReynolds, C. and Cox, R. (1970) Motivation and personality. New York, NY: Harper and Row.

Mavridou, P., Dimitriou, V., Manataki, A., Arnaoutoglou, E. and Papadopoulos, G. (2013) Patient's anxiety and fear of anesthesia: effect of gender, age, education, and previous experience of anesthesia. A survey of 400 patients. *Journal of Anesthesia,* 27: 104–108.

May, C. P., Rahhal, T., Berry, E. M. and Leighton, E. A. (2005) Aging, source memory, and emotion. *Psychology and Aging,* 20(4): 571–578.

Maykovich, M. K. (1978) Social constraints in eating patterns among the obese and overweight. *Social Problems,* 453–460.

Mayou, R. A., Black, J. and Bryant, B. (2000) Unconsciousness, amnesia and psychiatric symptoms following road traffic accident injury. *The British Journal of Psychiatry,* 177: 540–545.

McCarley, R. W. and Hobson, J. A. (1979) The form of dreams and the biology of sleep. *Handbook of dreams: research, theories and applications,* pp. 76–130.

McCrone, P., Sharpe, M., Chalder, T., Knapp, M., Johnson, A. L., Goldsmith, K. A. and White, P. D. (2012) Adaptive pacing, cognitive behaviour therapy, graded exercise, and specialist medical care for chronic fatigue syndrome: a cost-effectiveness analysis. *PloS one,* 7: e40808.

McIntosh, D. N. (1996) Facial feedback hypotheses: evidence, implications, and directions. *Motivation and Emotion,* 20: 121–147.

McKeown, T. (1979) *The Role of Medicine.* Oxford, UK: Blackwell.

McKeown, T. (2014) *The role of medicine: dream, mirage, or nemesis?* Princeton, NJ: Princeton University Press.

Melinder, C., Udumyan, R., Hiyoshi, A., Brummer, R. and Montgomery, S. (2015) Decreased stress resilience in young men significantly increases the risk of subsequent peptic ulcer disease – a prospective study of 233 093 men in Sweden. *Alimentary Pharmacology and Therapeutics,* 41: 1005–1015.

Melzack, R. and Wall, P. D. (1967) Pain mechanisms: a new theory. *Survey of Anesthesiology,* 11: 89–90.

Milgrim, S (1963) Behavioural Study of Obedience. *The Journal of Abnormal and Social Psychology,* 67 (4): 371–378.

Miller, G. A. (1956) The magical number seven, plus or minus two: some limits on our capacity for processing information. *Psychological Review,* 63: 81–97.

Miller, N. E. (1951) Illustrated by the development of a theory of conflict behavior. *Journal of Personality,* 20: 82–100.

Mischel, W. and Moore, B. (1973) Effects of attention to symbolically presented rewards on self-control. *Journal of Personality and Social Psychology,* 28 (2): 172–179.

Mishra, S. I., Scherer, R. W., Snyder, C., Geigle, P. M., Berlanstein, D. R. and Topaloglu, O. (2012) Exercise interventions on health-related quality of life for people with cancer during active treatment. *Cochrane Database of Systematic Reviews* August 15; (8): CD008465.

Miyake, A., Friedman, N. P., Emerson, M. J., Witzki, A. H., Howerter, A. and Wager, T. D. (2000) The unity and diversity of executive functions and their contributions to complex "frontal lobe" tasks: a latent variable analysis. *Cognitive Psychology,* 41: 49–100.

Monk, C., Fifer, W. P., Myers, M. M., Sloan, R. P., Trien, L. and Hurtado, A. (2000) Maternal stress responses and anxiety during pregnancy: effects on fetal heart rate. *Developmental Psychobiology*, 36: 67–77.

Moos, R. H. and Schaefer, J. A. (1984) 'The crisis of physical illness' in R. Moos (Ed.) *Coping with Physical Illness 2: new perspectives.* New York, NY: Plenum.

Motamedi, M. H. K. (2012) Thinking outside of the box. *Trauma Monthly*, 17: 217–218.

Mozaffarian, D., Benjamin, E. J., Go, A. S., Arnett, D. K., Blaha, M. J., Cushman, M., Das, S. R., De Ferranti, S., Després, J.-P. and Fullerton, H. J. (2016) Executive summary: heart disease and stroke statistics – 2016 update: a report from the American Heart Association. *Circulation*, 133: 447–454.

Mufune, P. (2015) Poverty and HIV/AIDS in Africa: specifying the connections. *Social Theory and Health*, 13: 1–29.

Mulder, G. (1986) The concept and measurement of mental effort. Energetics and human information processing. Dordrecht, NL: Springer-Verlag.

Mulder, E., De Medina, P. R., Huizink, A., Van Den Bergh, B., Buitelaar, J. and Visser, G. (2002) Prenatal maternal stress: effects on pregnancy and the (unborn) child. *Early Human Development*, 70: 3–14.

Murphy, L. R. (1996) Stress management in work settings: a critical review of the health effects. *American Journal of Health Promotion*, 11: 112–135.

Murray, J., Ehlers, A. and Mayou, R. A. (2002) Dissociation and post-traumatic stress disorder: two prospective studies of road traffic accident survivors. *The British Journal of Psychiatry*, 180: 363–368.

Muse, M. B. (1925) *A textbook of psychology*. Philadelphia, PA and London: W. B. Saunders Company.

Muse, M. B. (1934) *A textbook of psychology* (3rd Ed.). Philadelphia, PA and London: W. B. Saunders Company.

Myers, D. G. (2004) *Exploring psychology*. New York, NY: Worth Publishers.

Nash, R. A. and Takarangi, M. K. (2011) Reconstructing alcohol-induced memory blackouts. *Memory*, 19: 566–573.

Neeman, E. and Ben-Eliyahu, S. (2013) Surgery and stress promote cancer metastasis: new outlooks on perioperative mediating mechanisms and immune involvement. *Brain, Behavior, and Immunity*, 30: S32-S40.

Nes, L. S. and Segerstrom, S. C. (2006) Dispositional optimism and coping: a meta-analytic review. *Personality and Social Psychology Review*, 10: 235–251.

Neugarten, B. L. and Havighurst, R. J. (1969) 'Disengagement reconsidered in a cross-national context', Chapter 22 in R. J. Havighurst, J. M. A. Munnichs, B.L. Neugarten and H. Thomae (Eds) *Adjustment to retirement.* Assen, NL: van Gorcum and Company, pp. 138–146.

Neumann, R. and Strack, F. (2000) "Mood contagion": the automatic transfer of mood between persons. *Journal of Personality and Social Psychology*, 79 (2): 211–223.

Nickerson, R. S. (1998) Confirmation bias: a ubiquitous phenomenon in many guises. *Review of General Psychology*, 2: 175.

Nieuwlaat, R., Wilczynski, N., Navarro, T., Hobson, N., Jeffery, R., Keepanasseril, A. ... Jack, S. (2014) Interventions for enhancing medication adherence. *Cochrane Database of Systematic Reviews*, 11.

Nilsson, U., Unosson, M. and Rawal, N. (2005) Stress reduction and analgesia in patients exposed to calming music postoperatively: a randomized controlled trial. *European Journal of Anaesthesiology*, 22(02), 96–102.

NMC (2010) Standards of proficiency for pre-registration nursing education. London: Nursing and Midwifery Council. Available at: http://www.nmc-uk.org/documents/standards/nmcstandardsofprofi iencyforpre_registrationnursingeducation.pdf (last accessed 10 April 2016).

NMC (2015) *The code: professional standards of practice and behaviour for nurses and midwives.* London: Nursing and Midwifery Council.

Nolen-Hoeksema, S., Frederickson, B., Loftus, G. and Lutz, C. (2014) *Atkinson & Hilgard's Introduction to Psychology* (16th Ed.). Andover, Hampshire, UK: Cengage Learning.

Odlum, D. M. (1952) *Psychology, the nurse and the patient* (1st Ed.). New York, NY: Philosophical Library.

O'Dougherty, M., Story, M. and Stang, J. (2006) Observations of parent-child co-shoppers in supermarkets: children's involvement in food selections, parental yielding, and refusal strategies. *Journal of Nutrition Education and Behavior*, 38: 183–188.

Ogden, J. (2012) *Health psychology.* Maidenhead, UK: Open University Press.

Olds, J. (1956) Pleasure centers in the brain. *Scientific American*, 195: 105–117.

Omlin, A., Blum, D., Wierecky, J., Haile, S. R., Ottery, F. D. and Strasser, F. (2013) Nutrition impact symptoms in advanced cancer patients: frequency and specific interventions, a case–control study. *Journal of Cachexia, Sarcopenia and Muscle*, 4: 55–61.

Orr, W. C. and Stahl, M. L. (1977) Sleep disturbances after open heart surgery. *The American Journal of Cardiology*, 39: 196–201.

O'Sullivan, E. (2015) Dealing with the difficult patient. *Annals of Emergency Medicine*, 66: 555–555.

Paley, J. (2014) Cognition and the compassion deficit: the social psychology of helping behaviour in nursing. *Nursing Philosophy*, 15: 274–287.

Papalia, D. E., Wendkos Old, S. and Duskin Feldman, R. (2004) *Human Development* (9th Ed.). New York, NY: McGraw-Hill.

Patel, A. (2013) Review: the role of inflammation in depression. *Psychiatria Danubina*, 25: S216–23.

Pavlov, I. P. (1906) The scientific investigation of the psychical faculties or processes in the higher animals. *Science*, 24: 613–619.

Penedo, F. J. and Dahn, J. R. (2005) Exercise and well-being: a review of mental and physical health benefits associated with physical activity. *Current Opinion in Psychiatry*, 18: 189–193.

Perry, B. D. (2008) 'Child maltreatment: a neurodevelopmental perspective on the role of trauma and neglect in psychopathology' in T. Beauchaine and S. P. Hinshaw (Eds) *Textbook of Child and Adolescent Psychopathology*, pp. 93–128.

Perry, B. D. and Szalavitz, M. (2007) *The boy who was raised as a dog and other stories from a child psychiatrist's notebook: what traumatized children can teach us about loss, love and healing.* New York, NY: Basic Books.

Peterson, D. I. (1967) Developing the difficult patient. *The American Journal of Nursing*, 67 (3): 522–525.

Petty, R. E. and Cacioppo, J. T. (1986) *Communication and persuasion: central and peripheral routes to attitude change*. New York, NY: Springer-Verlag.

Phelvin, A. (2014) Winterbourne View hospital and the social psychology of abuse. *Learning Disability Practice*, 17, 10, 25–29.

Piaget, J. (1959) *The language and thought of the child*. Hove, UK: Psychology Press.

Piaget, J. (1976) *Piaget's theory*. Dordrecht, NL: Springer.

Piaget, J. and Inhelder, B. (1969) *The psychology of the child*. New York, NY: Basic Books.

Plomin, R., Defries, J. C., Knopik, V. S. and Neiderheiser, J. (2013) *Behavioral genetics*. Palgrave Macmillan.

Plsek, P. E. and Wilson, T. (2001) Complexity science: complexity, leadership, and management in health-care organisations. *BMJ: British Medical Journal*, 323: 746–749.

Plutchik, R. (1980) *Emotion: a psychoevolutionary synthesis*. New York, NY: Harper and Row.

Polit, D. F. and Beck, C. T. (2013) *Essentials of nursing research: appraising evidence for nursing practice*. London: Lippincott Williams & Wilkins.

Ponchel, A., Bombois, S., Bordet, R. and Hénon, H. (2015) Factors associated with poststroke fatigue: a systematic review. *Stroke Research and Treatment*, doi: 10.1155/2015/347920.

Ponsford, J. L., Parcell, D. L., Sinclair, K. L., Roper, M. and Rajaratnam, S. M. (2013) Changes in sleep patterns following traumatic brain injury: a controlled study. *Neurorehabilitation and Neural Repair*, 27: 613–621.

Powell, N., Tarr, A. and Sheridan, J. F. (2013) Psychosocial stress and inflammation in cancer. *Brain, Behavior, and Immunity*, 30: S41-S47.

Prochaska, J. O. and Di Clemente, C. C. (1986) *Toward a comprehensive model of change*. New York, NY: Plenum Press.

Raczynski, J. M. and DiClemente, R. J. (2013) *Handbook of health promotion and disease prevention*. New York, NY: Springer Science + Business Media.

Ramaekers, S. and Suissa, J. (2012) 'Good Enough Parenting?' Chapter 4 in S. Ramaekers and J. Suissa *The Claims of Parenting*. Dordrecht, NL: Springer.

Rana, D. and Upton, D. (2013) *Psychology for nurses*. London: Routledge.

Reason, J. (1990) *Human error*. Cambridge, UK: Cambridge University Press.

Reason, J. (1993) 'Managing the management risk: new approaches to organisational safety' in B. Wilpert and T. Qvale (Eds) *Reliability and safety in hazardous work systems*. Hove, UK: Lawrence Erlbaum Associates, pp. 7–22.

Reason, J., Hollnagel, E. and Paries, J. (2006) Revisiting the «Swiss cheese» model of accidents. *Journal of Clinical Engineering*, 27: 110–115.

Roach, M. S. (2013) 'Caring: the human mode of being' in M. C. Smith, M. C. Turkel and Z. Robinson-Wolf (Eds) *Caring in nursing classics: an essential resource*. New York, NY: Springer (pp. 165–179).

Robertson, I. (2012) *The winner effect: how power affects your brain.* London: Bloomsbury.

Robinson, E., Thomas, J., Aveyard, P. and Higgs, S. (2014) What everyone else is eating: a systematic review and meta-analysis of the effect of informational eating norms on eating behavior. *Journal of the Academy of Nutrition and Dietetics,* 114: 414–429.

Robinson, R. G. and Jorge, R. E. (2015) Post-stroke depression: a review. *American Journal of Psychiatry,* 173 (3): 221–231.

Rodin, J. and Langer, E. J. (1977) Long-term effects of a control-relevant intervention with the institutionalized aged. *Journal of Personality and Social Psychology,* 35 (12): 897–902.

Rogers, C. R. (1951) *Client-centered therapy: its current practice, implications, and theory.* London: Constable.

Rolfe, G., Jasper, M. and Freshwater, D. (2010) *Critical reflection in practice: generating knowledge for care* (2nd Ed.). Hampshire, UK: Palgrave Macmillan.

Ross, C. A. and Goldner, E. M. (2009) Stigma, negative attitudes and discrimination towards mental illness within the nursing profession: a review of the literature. *Journal of Psychiatric and Mental Health Nursing,* 16: 558–567.

Rydon-Grange, M. (2015) 'What's Psychology got to do with it?' Applying psychological theory to understanding failures in modern healthcare settings. *Journal of Medical Ethics,* medethics–2015–102922.

Sadja, J. and Mills, P. J. (2013) Effects of yoga interventions on fatigue in cancer patients and survivors: a systematic review of randomized controlled trials. *Explore: The Journal of Science and Healing,* 9: 232–243.

Saunders, L. E., Green, J. M., Petticrew, M. P., Steinbach, R. and Roberts, H. (2013) What are the health benefits of active travel? A systematic review of trials and cohort studies. *PLoS One,* 8, e69912.

Schacter, D. L. (1999) The seven sins of memory: insights from psychology and cognitive neuroscience. *American Psychologist,* 54 (3): 182–203.

Schacter, D. L. and Addis, D. R. (2007) The cognitive neuroscience of constructive memory: remembering the past and imagining the future. *Philosophical Transactions of the Royal Society B: Biological Sciences,* 362: 773–786.

Schachter, S. and Singer, J. (1962) Cognitive, social, and physiological determinants of emotional state. *Psychological Review,* 69: 379–399.

Schaufeli, W. B., Leiter, M. P. and Maslach, C. (2009) Burnout: 35 years of research and practice. *Career Development International,* 14: 204–220.

Scheier, M. F. and Carver, C. S. (1993) On the power of positive thinking: the benefits of being optimistic. *Current Directions in Psychological Science,* 2: 26–30.

Schramm, W. (1971) 'The nature of communication between humans' in W. Schramm and D. E. Roberts (Eds) *The process and effects of mass communication.* Urbana: University of Illinois Press, pp. 3–53.

Schwartz, S. H. and Clausen, G. T. (1970) Responsibility, norms, and helping in an emergency. *Journal of Personality and Social Psychology,* 16 (2): 299–310.

Schwender, D., Kaiser, A., Klasing, S., Peter, K. and Pöppel, E. (1994) Midlatency auditory evoked potentials and explicit and implicit memory in patients undergoing cardiac surgery. *Anesthesiology,* 80: 493–501.

Seligman, M. E. (1971) Phobias and preparedness. *Behavior Therapy*, 2: 307–320.

Seligman, M. E. (2011) *Learned optimism: how to change your mind and your life.* New York, NY: Vintage Books (Random House).

Seligman, M. E. and Csikszentmihalyi, M. (2000) *Positive psychology: an introduction.* American Psychological Association. *American Psychologist*, 55 (1): 5–14.

Selye, H. (1956) *The stress of life.* New York, NY: McGraw-Hill.

Sherif, M., Harvey, O., White, B., Hood, W. and Sherif, C. (1961) *Intergroup cooperation and conflict: the robbers' cave experiment.* Norman, OK: University of Oklahoma Book Exchange.

Shimizu, M., Johnson, K. and Wansink, B. (2014) In good company. The effect of an eating companion's appearance on food intake. *Appetite*, 83: 263–268.

Skinner, B. F. (1938) *The behavior of organisms: an experimental analysis.* New York, NY: Appleton-Century-Crofts, Inc.

Skinner, B. F. (1972) *Beyond freedom and dignity.* New York, NY: Bantam Books.

Skinner, B. F. and Hayes, J. (1976) *Walden Two.* New York, NY: Macmillan.

Sklar, L. S. and Anisman, H. (1981) Stress and cancer. *Psychological Bulletin*, 89 (3): 369–406.

Slade, A., Cohen, L. J., Sadler, L. S. and Miller, M. (2009) 'The psychology and psychopathology of pregnancy' Chapter 2 in Charles H. Zeanah Jr. (Ed.) *The Handbook of Infant Mental Health*, pp. 22–39.

Smit, C. (2015) Theories and models of grief: applications to professional practice. *Whitireia Nursing and Health Journal*: 33.

Smith, J., Forster, A., Young, J. and Stroke, C. G. F. I. P. A. (2009) Cochrane review: information provision for stroke patients and their caregivers. *Clinical Rehabilitation*, 23: 195–206.

Smith-Miller, C. A., Shaw-Kokot, J., Curro, B. and Jones, C. B. (2014) An integrative review: fatigue among nurses in acute care settings. *Journal of Nursing Administration*, 44: 487–494.

Soderstrom, M., Dolbier, C., Leiferman, J. and Steinhardt, M. (2000) The relationship of hardiness, coping strategies, and perceived stress to symptoms of illness. *Journal of Behavioral Medicine*, 23: 311–328.

Spencer, S. J., Steele, C. M. and Quinn, D. M. (1999) Stereotype threat and women's math performance. *Journal of Experimental Social Psychology*, 35: 4–28.

Stamenov, M. and Gallese, V. (2002) *Mirror neurons and the evolution of brain and language.* Amsterdam, NL: John Benjamins Publishing.

Staud, R., Mokthech, M., Price, D. D. and Robinson, M. E. (2015) Evidence for sensitized fatigue pathways in patients with chronic fatigue syndrome. *Pain*, 156: 750–759.

Steblay, N. M. (1992) A meta-analytic review of the weapon focus effect. *Law and Human Behavior*, 16: 413.

Steele, C. M. (1988) The psychology of self-affirmation: sustaining the integrity of the self. *Advances in Experimental Social Psychology*, 21: 261–302.

Steele, C. M. and Aronson, J. (1995) Stereotype threat and the intellectual test performance of African Americans. *Journal of Personality and Social Psychology*, 69: 797–811.

Steele, C. M., Spencer, S. J. and Aronson, J. (2002) Contending with group image: the psychology of stereotype and social identity threat. *Advances in Experimental Social Psychology*, 34: 379–440.

Steptoe, A. and Kivimäki, M. (2013) Stress and cardiovascular disease: an update on current knowledge. *Annual Review of Public Health*, 34: 337–354.

Stern, D. N. (2010) *Forms of vitality: exploring dynamic experience in psychology, the arts, psychotherapy, and development.* Oxford University Press.

Sternberg, R. J. (1986) A triangular theory of love. *Psychological Review*, 93 (2): 119–135.

Stroebe, M. and Schut, H. (1999) The dual process model of coping with bereavement: rationale and description. *Death Studies*, 23: 197–224.

Stroebe, M., Schut, H. and Stroebe, W. (1998) 'Trauma and grief: a comparative analysis' in J. Harvey (Ed.) *Perspectives on loss: a sourcebook.* Philadelphia, PA: Brunner/Mazel, pp. 81–96.

Swaab, D. (1991) Brain aging and Alzheimer's disease, "wear and tear" versus "use it or lose it". *Neurobiology of Aging*, 12: 317–324.

Sykes, J. and Javidnia, H. (2013) A contemporary review of the management of the difficult patient. *JAMA facial plastic surgery*, 15: 81–84.

Takase, M., Maude, P. and Manias, E. (2006) Impact of the perceived public image of nursing on nurses' work behaviour. *Journal of Advanced Nursing*, 53: 333–343.

Tangney, J. P. and Fisher, K. W. (1995) *Self-conscious emotions: the psychology of shame, guilt, embarrassment, and pride.* New York, NY: Guilford Press.

Taylor, S. E. (1983) Adjustment to threatening events: a theory of cognitive adaptation. *American Psychologist*, 38 (11): 1161–1173.

Taylor, S. E., Lichtman, R. R. and Wood, J. V. (1984) Attributions, beliefs about control, and adjustment to breast cancer. *Journal of Personality and Social Psychology*, 46 (3): 489–502.

Thomas, A. G., Dennis, A., Bandettini, P. A. and Johansen-Berg, H. (2012) The effects of aerobic activity on brain structure. *Frontiers in Psychology*, 3.

Thompson, A., Hollis, C. and Richards, D. (2003) Authoritarian parenting attitudes as a risk for conduct problems. *European Child & Adolescent Psychiatry*, 12: 84–91.

Thorndike, E. L. (1927) The law of effect. *The American Journal of Psychology*, 39 (1): 212–222.

Timmins, F. and de Vries, J. M. (2014) Nurses are not bystanders: a response to Paley. *Nurse Education Today*, 34(10): 1269–1334.

Todorovic, D. (2008) Gestalt principles. *Scholarpedia*, 3 (12): 5345.

Tooby, J. and Cosmides, L. (1990) The past explains the present: emotional adaptations and the structure of ancestral environments. *Ethology and Sociobiology*, 11: 375–424.

Tooby, J. and Cosmides, L. (2008) 'The evolutionary psychology of the emotions and their relationship to internal regulatory variables' in M. Lewis, J. M. Haviland-Jones and L. Feldman Barrett (Eds) *Handbook of emotions*, (3rd Ed.). New York, NY: The Guildford Press.

Trivers, R. L. (1971) The evolution of reciprocal altruism. *Quarterly Review of Biology*, 46 (1): 35–57.

Trivers, R. (2006) 'Reciprocal altruism: 30 years later' in P. M. Kappeler and C. P. van Schaik (Eds) *Cooperation in Primates and Humans*. Berlin Heidelberg: Springer-Verlag.

Tulving, E. (2002) Episodic memory: from mind to brain. *Annual Review of Psychology*, 53: 1–25.

Upton, D. and Thirlaway, K. (2010) *Promoting healthy behaviour: a practical guide for nursing and healthcare professionals*. Harlow, UK: Pearson Education Limited.

Urquhart, D. M., Phyomaung, P. P., Dubowitz, J., Fernando, S., Wluka, A. E., Raajmaakers, P., Wang, Y. and Cicuttini, F. M. (2015) Are cognitive and behavioural factors associated with knee pain? A systematic review. *Seminars in Arthritis and Rheumatism*, Feb; 44(4): 445–55.

Van der Kolk, B. A. and McFarlane, A. C. (2012) *Traumatic stress: the effects of overwhelming experience on mind, body, and society*. Guilford Press.

Van der Kolk, B. A., Pelcovitz, D., Roth, S., Mandel, F., McFarlane, A. and Herman, J. L. (1996) Dissociation, somatization, and affect dysregulation: the complexity of adaptation to trauma. *American Journal of Psychiatry*, 153: 83–93.

Vargas, M. A. D. O. and Ramos, F. R. S. (2011) Responsibility in health care: regarding the time we live as intensive care nurses. *Revista da Escola de Enfermagem da USP*, 45: 876–883.

Veehof, M., Trompetter, H., Bohlmeijer, E. and Schreurs, K. (2016) Acceptance- and mindfulness-based interventions for The treatment of chronic pain: a meta-analytic review. *Cognitive Behaviour Therapy*, 45(1): 5–31.

Vetter, D., Barth, J., Uyulmaz, S., Uyulmaz, S., Vonlanthen, R., Belli, G. ... Clavien, P.-A. (2015) Effects of art on surgical patients: a systematic review and meta-analysis. *Annals of Surgery*, 262(5): 704–713.

Vissing, Y. M., Straus, M. A., Gelles, R. J. and Harrop, J. W. (1991) Verbal aggression by parents and psychosocial problems of children. *Child Abuse & Neglect*, 15: 223–238.

Volker, S., Keller, H., Lohaus, A., Cappenberg, M. and Chasiotis, A. (1999) Maternal interactive behaviour in early infancy and later attachment. *International Journal of Behavioral Development*, 23: 921–936.

Vygotsky, L. (1978) Interaction between learning and development. *Readings on the Development of Children*, 23(3): 34–41.

Wahrendorf, M., Ribet, C., Zins, M., Goldberg, M. and Siegrist, J. (2010) Perceived reciprocity in social exchange and health functioning in early old age: prospective findings from the GAZEL study. *Aging & Mental Health*, 14: 425–432.

Walker, J., Payne, S., Jarrett, N. and Ley, T. (2012) *Psychology for nurses and the caring professions*. New York, NY: McGraw-Hill International.

Walsh, K. and Kowanko, I. (2002) Nurses' and patients' perceptions of dignity. *International Journal of Nursing Practice*. 8: 143–151.

Walton, G. M., Murphy, M. C. and Ryan, A. M. (2015) Stereotype threat in organizations: implications for equity and performance. *Annual Review of Organizational Psychology and Organizational Behavior*, 2: 523–550.

Ward, J. (2010) *The Student's Guide to Cognitive Neuroscience* (2nd Ed.). Hove and New York: Psychology Press (Taylor and Francis Group).

Wason, P. C. and Johnson-Laird, P. N. (1972) *Psychology of reasoning: structure and content.* Cambridge, MA: Harvard University Press.

Watanabe, N., Stewart, R., Jenkins, R., Bhugra, D. K. and Furukawa, T. A. (2008) The epidemiology of chronic fatigue, physical illness, and symptoms of common mental disorders: a cross-sectional survey from the second British National Survey of Psychiatric Morbidity. *Journal of Psychosomatic Research*, 64: 357–362.

Watson, J. B. and Rayner, R. (1920) Conditioned emotional reactions. *Journal of Experimental Psychology*, 3 (1): 1–14.

Watt-Watson, J., Garfinkel, P., Gallop, R., Stevens, B. and Streiner, D. (2000). The impact of nurses' empathic responses on patients' pain management in acute care. *Nursing Research*, 49(4): 191–200.

Weiner, B. (1988) Attribution theory and attributional therapy: some theoretical observations and suggestions. *British Journal of Clinical Psychology*, 27: 99–104.

Weinreb, L., Wehler, C., Perloff, J., Scott, R., Hosmer, D., Sagor, L. and Gundersen, C. (2002) Hunger: its impact on children's health and mental health. *Pediatrics*, 110: e41-e41.

Weinstein, B. E. and Ventry, I. M. (1982) Hearing impairment and social isolation in the elderly. *Journal of Speech, Language, and Hearing Research*, 25: 593–599.

Weinstein, T. L. and Li, X. (2015) The relationship between stress and clinical outcomes for persons living with HIV/AIDS: a systematic review of the global literature. *AIDS Care.* 28(2): 160–9.

Weiten, W. (2010) *Psychology: Themes and Variations (briefer version)* (8th Int. Ed.) Belmont, CA: Wadsworth Cengage Learning.

Wertheimer, M. (1923) Laws of organization in perceptual forms. *A source book of Gestalt psychology*. London, UK: Routledge & Kegan Paul.

Westbrook, J. I., Duffield, C., Li, L. and Creswick, N. J. (2011) How much time do nurses have for patients? A longitudinal study quantifying hospital nurses' patterns of task time distribution and interactions with health professionals. *BMC Health Services Research*, 11: 319.

Whiteford, H. A., Degenhardt, L., Rehm, J., Baxter, A. J., Ferrari, A. J., Erskine, H. E., Charlson, F. J., Norman, R. E., Flaxman, A. D. and Johns, N. (2013) Global burden of disease attributable to mental and substance use disorders: findings from the Global Burden of Disease Study 2010. *The Lancet*, 382: 1575–1586.

WHO (2006) *Constitution of the World Health Organization.* Basic Documents, Supplement, October 2006. Geneva: World Health Organisation (WHO).

Williams, A., Eccleston, C. and Morley, S. (2012) Psychological therapies for the management of chronic pain (excluding headache) in adults. *Cochrane Database Syst Rev*, 11.

Wills, T. A. (1978) Perceptions of clients by professional helpers. *Psychological Bulletin*, 85 (5): 968–1000.

Winstanley, S. and Whittington, R. (2004) Aggression towards health care staff in a UK general hospital: variation among professions and departments. *Journal of Clinical Nursing*, 13(1): 3–10.

Wood, D., Bruner, J. S. and Ross, G. (1976) The role of tutoring in problem solving. *Journal of Child Psychology and Psychiatry*, 17(2): 89–100.

Yerkes, R. M. and Dodson, J. D. (1908) The relation of strength of stimulus to rapidity of habit-formation. *Journal of Comparative Neurology and Psychology*, 18, 459–482.

Yoder, E. A. (2010) Compassion fatigue in nurses. *Applied Nursing Research*, 23(4): 191–197.

Zedelius, C. M. and Schooler, J. W. (2015) Mind wandering "Ahas" versus mindful reasoning: alternative routes to creative solutions. *Frontiers in Psychology*, 6: 834.

Zerwekh, J. and Garneau, A. Z. (2014) *Nursing today: transition and trends* (8th Ed.). St Louis, MO: Elsevier Health Sciences.

Zimbardo, P. G., Haney, C., Banks, W. C. and Jaffe, D. (1974) 'The psychology of imprisonment: privation, power, and pathology' in Z. Rubin (Ed.) *Doing Unto Others: Explorations in Social Behavior.* Englewood Cliffs, NJ: Prentice-Hall, pp. 61–73.

Zwi, M., Jones, H., Thorgaard, C., York, A. and Dennis, J. A. (2011) *Parent training interventions for Attention Deficit Hyperactivity Disorder (ADHD) in children aged 5 to 18 years.* London: The Cochrane Library.

Index